Why Are We Still Getting HIV?

Teens Respond to the AIDS Epidemic

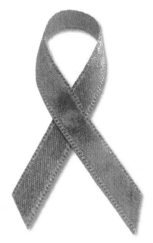

By Youth Communication

Edited by Laura Longhine

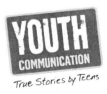

YOUTH
COMMUNICATION
True Stories by Teens

Why Are We Still Getting HIV?

EXECUTIVE EDITORS
Keith Hefner and Laura Longhine

CONTRIBUTING EDITORS
Tamar Rothenberg, Hope Vanderberg, Marie Glancy, Philip Kay,
Al Desetta, Andrea Estepa, Clarence Haynes, Katia Hetter,
Kendra Hurley, Nora McCarthy, and Alexandra Ringe

LAYOUT & DESIGN
Efrain Reyes, Jr. and Jeff Faerber

PRODUCTION
Stephanie Liu

COVER ART
YC Art Dept.

For reprint information, please contact Youth Communication.

ISBN 978-1-935552-37-6

Second, Expanded Edition

Printed in the United States of America

Youth Communication ®
New York, New York
www.youthcomm.org

Catalog Item #YD37-1

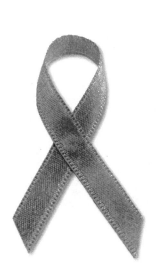

Table of Contents

Contents

Suffering in Silence

Twenty Years Living Positive

Acting Is My Activism

My Dad Has HIV

Too Big a Risk

Contents

Using the Book

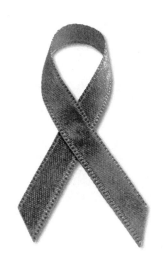

Introduction

By Adam Wacholder

It's been almost three decades since the first cases of HIV/AIDS were reported. So why exactly are people still getting this disease? Are the viruses getting bigger? Have they acquired new abilities through extraterrestrial cross-breeding? Maybe they're becoming more efficient killing machines by using the art of kung-fu!

Actually, none of these ideas are true, and that's why we're here. Our mission in this book is to give you the latest facts on HIV/AIDS, the truth about how it's affecting our lives, and strategies for how to protect yourself.

Here's a fact to ponder. In 2007, more than 559,000 people in the United States died from cancer. Meanwhile, an estimated 14,561 Americans lost their battle with AIDS. When I first saw these statistics, I was confused. If almost 40 times as many people in this country are dying from cancer than AIDS, why are we making such a big deal over AIDS?

Then I figured it out. Cancer is a condition that attacks out of the blue and there's no solid means of prevention. Eating broccoli might help, but don't count on it. AIDS, on the other hand, has the most solid method of prevention known to man and woman: wear a condom if you're having sex, and if you're not mature enough to, then just don't have sex at all. (I won't even go near the issue of sharing hypodermic needles. I hope you're not shooting up with heroin.)

So if HIV/AIDS is preventable, what's stopping us from eliminating this disease?

We teens think we're invincible. We think nothing bad can ever happen to us, and as a 17-year-old, I admit I feel this way too. But that's exactly the mentality that's led people under age 25 to make up half of the world's brand-new HIV patients. It's also the reason why five more young people are infected every minute.

Several of the stories in this book show how, even when we know the facts, we sometimes still put ourselves at risk by having unprotected sex. For example, one writer has sex without a condom after getting drunk at a party. "My good judgment had disappeared due to the happy, careless feeling that came with the liquor," she writes. "As soon as I sobered up, I realized I might have exposed myself to a deadly disease, and I was furious with myself."

Another problem is our lack of communication about HIV. If you're sexually active, have you ever asked your partner how many people he or she has had sex with, or if they've ever had unprotected sex or used IV drugs? Have you ever felt too uncomfortable to ask a partner to wear a condom?

Several teens in this book share how they've handled those difficult discussions with partners, or taken other sometimes uncomfortable steps to protect themselves, like getting an HIV test, buying condoms, or reaching out for help.

Since the disease first surfaced, there have been major advances in treatment. Unlike some of the people in these stories, who contracted the disease early on and died relatively quickly, people with HIV can now live with it for many years, even decades. But there's still no cure. Many of these writers share the pain of watching a loved one get sick or losing them to AIDS. Others who've been infected themselves write about how the disease has changed their lives. We hope their stories will help you think seriously about the risks you take and how best to stay safe. It's time for teens to step up and stop the spread of HIV.

Adam was in high school when he wrote this story.

In the following stories, names have been changed: *What If...?*, *Keeping Quiet*, *My Uncle Died of AIDS*, *Date With Destiny*, *My Dad Has HIV*, and *Too Big A Risk*.

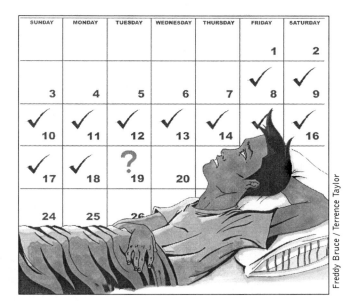

SUNDAY	MONDAY	TUESDAY	WEDNESDAY	THURSDAY	FRIDAY	SATURDAY
					1	2
3	4	5	6	7	✓ 8	✓ 9
✓ 10	✓ 11	✓ 12	✓ 13	✓ 14	✓	✓ 16
✓ 17	✓ 18	? 19	20			
24	25	26				

Freddy Bruce / Terrence Taylor

What If...?

By Anonymous

I was in health class one day last spring, expecting another boring lecture on drugs and alcohol, or smoking, or pregnancy, when a tall, balding white man with a mustache and a funny smile came into the room. Some of the kids knew who he was and called out, "Hey, Dave."

"Hey," he replied, with a wave.

Dave is the health and drug prevention counselor at my school. He was in my class to conduct a lesson on HIV/AIDS. I wasn't interested in AIDS. I figured since I didn't have it and neither did my friends, why should it bother me? But as Dave began to talk, the facts came out: people can have the AIDS virus and not even know it.

He said the disease is killing millions of people around the world. He explained how HIV, the virus that causes AIDS, is transmitted through oral, anal, and vaginal sex, and also through hypodermic needles.

But after I heard the part about "sexually transmitted orally," I stopped listening and drifted back in my mind to the previous summer.

It was raining. I was at this girl's house. Her parents were still at work and her sister was sleeping down the hall, so we had to be quiet.

We performed oral sex on each other. We never really had a chance to go all the way—we stopped when it started to thunder outside because we were afraid her sister would wake up and catch us. But apparently we did go far enough to put ourselves at risk for AIDS. We hadn't used any protection. The word "condom" never even came up.

I wasn't interested in AIDS. I figured since I didn't have it and neither did my friends, why should it bother me?

All of a sudden the bell rang and I found myself sitting there in health class, somewhat dazed. On the board was Dave's name and room number. I felt I had to find out more about AIDS, so I went to his office to see him that afternoon.

I told him about my first encounter with unprotected oral sex the previous summer. Dave said that it was possible to get infected that way and said that if I was HIV-positive, the sooner I knew the better, because there was treatment for it which could help me. He told me to take some time to think about what he'd said and whether or not I wanted to take the HIV test. Then he gave me some numbers I could call for information about where to go.

I waited a couple of weeks and I finally decided to go through with it. If anyone could get this disease from unprotected sex, then why not me? I wanted to know.

I called up the AIDS hotline and they gave me the phone number of the anonymous testing center nearest to my house. I called up and made an appointment. I didn't even have to give them my name. They gave me a number instead and told me when to come in and how to get there.

The center was in a dirty neighborhood. There were bums on the sidewalks, graffiti on the buildings, and garbage on the streets. The center itself was in an old school. "If it looks the same on the inside," I thought, "I don't want to go through with the test."

But inside it was reasonably clean. There were other people waiting and a man behind a desk. "I have an appointment to take an HIV test," I told him.

He said to have a seat. I wasn't really sure if all the other people were there for the same reason or not. I sat down and thought to myself, "What am I doing? Why am I here? What if I'm HIV-positive?" I was still kind of confused, but I knew it was my responsibility to my family, friends, and myself to find out if I was infected.

Finally this short, middle-aged lady came into the room and told me to follow her. We went into a small room in the back of the building with a desk and a couple of chairs. The room had posters on the wall with information about HIV and AIDS and there was a bowl of condoms on one of the tables.

"I'm Lydia" she said.

I didn't tell her my name. I didn't have to. Lydia asked me why I was there.

"I had oral sex, and I wanted to know if I have HIV." I knew it was one of the least likely way to catch AIDS sexually, but there was always that risk.

I was kind of uncomfortable at first. I didn't know what to expect. But Lydia was very considerate. "When was the last time you had sexual contact?" she asked.

"About 10 months ago," I said.

Lydia explained that this was good because infections show up on the test six months after you've been infected.

"What are you going to do if you're positive?" she asked.

"Either way, I'm going to have to change my ways," I said. "If I'm negative, then I have to be responsible and stay that way. If I'm positive, then I'll be open about it. I'll tell my family and friends." In my mind I was thinking that I'd find the courage to be a role model. I wanted to let people know that AIDS is still infecting people.

Lydia wrote down what I was telling her. Then she told me about syphilis and other sexually transmitted diseases. She showed me some pictures of people's genital warts. It was really disgusting. She put everything she had written down into a folder and made an appointment for me to come back in two weeks to find out my results.

Then Lydia directed me to another room to take the test. On my way out, I grabbed as many pamphlets as I could. I wanted as much information on AIDS as I could carry. I grabbed a couple of condoms too. If I did have sex again, I wanted to make sure I was protected.

A nurse told me to have a seat, take off my jacket, and roll up my sleeve. As she brought out the needle she said, "This won't hurt."

"I'm not scared of needles," I told her and I watched as she drew two dark red vials of blood from my arm.

After that, my only concern was getting to the subway station and home. I felt so weird. What if I ran into someone I knew?

When I got back to my neighborhood, I stopped at McDonald's to get something to eat. But the line was so long I decided not to wait. As I turned to leave, all the AIDS pamphlets fell out of my notebook and onto the floor. I was embarrassed. I quickly I got on my knees and tried to pick everything up. I didn't hear anybody say anything, but my heart was beating fast and it felt like everyone was staring at me, wondering, "Why does he have all of those pamphlets on AIDS?"

On the way home, I ran into a friend I hadn't spoken to for a long time. "What's been going on with you lately?" she asked, but I didn't say much. I couldn't bring myself to tell her what I was going through and where I had just been.

The only person I trusted was Dave. He told me more about AIDS. I learned about how the virus is transmitted and what happens to your body when you have HIV.

At school, I tried concentrating on other things besides the test. I found I actually wanted to study just so I could take my mind off of the two week wait.

But every night before I went to sleep I thought about it again. I had so many questions: What would I actually do when I got my results? Would I really be open about it? Would I fool around again without using a condom?

It gave me such a headache. I was driving myself crazy thinking about what I'd done. I lost my appetite and I even lost touch with some of my friends. I realized I was too young for this and, no matter what the results, I didn't want to go through all this worry ever again.

I couldn't bring myself to tell her what I was going through and where I had just been.

After the two weeks, I went back to the center and saw Lydia. We went straight into her office. It was weird because at that moment, I wasn't worried. There had to be a bright side to all this and I was determined to find it.

Lydia got out my folder from a filing cabinet and we sat down. She put the folder on the table and asked me some questions. I can't remember what she was saying because my mind was completely focused on the folder. Finally she opened it up and in dark bold lettering was the word "NEGATIVE."

Lydia said something else, but I couldn't pay attention. I was thinking about everything I went through—how I ran around this unfamiliar neighborhood, how embarrassed I felt at McDonald's, and how I'd kept all this from my family and friends.

I only asked Lydia one question: "How many times is the blood tested?" I wanted to be sure.

"Three times," she said. I felt relieved. She got me out of her office pretty quickly after that, but I understood. Who knows, maybe her next appointment was with someone who'd find out they had tested positive for HIV.

For more information on HIV-testing, see p. 116.

The author was in high school when he wrote this story.

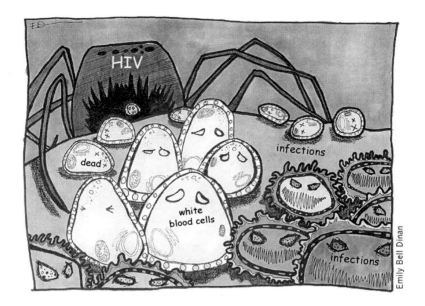

Emily Bell Dinan

How HIV Works

By Zaineb Nadeem

During a discussion about HIV/AIDS in my science class during freshman year, I asked my teacher, "What can we do to get rid of the virus?"

"We don't have a cure for HIV/AIDS," she answered. "It's fatal."

I was stunned to hear that they don't have a cure for this terrible thing. It was hot that day, but I remember shivering from the fear of getting it. We'd just learned about how the virus kills the immune system, and I didn't want to die like that.

But after studying HIV in class and doing research on my own, I realized that we can all understand the virus and protect ourselves from it if we have the right information. Here's what you need to know:

What is HIV/AIDS?

HIV is a virus (it stands for human immunodeficiency virus) that attacks the immune system, making it harder for your body to fight off infections. AIDS (acquired immunodeficiency syndrome) is the last stage of having HIV.

When a person has HIV in her or his body, it doesn't mean that the person has AIDS right away. It takes time for HIV to turn into AIDS. In some people it might take a year, in others it might take 10 or more years. But it always develops into AIDS at some point.

How HIV Spreads

HIV spreads through direct contact with an infected person's blood, semen (including pre-cum), vaginal fluid, or breast milk. You can get HIV through vaginal, oral, or anal sex with an HIV-positive person and by sharing needles (to inject drugs) with an HIV-positive person. (HIV-positive means that a person has the virus in his or her blood.)

An estimated one million people in the U.S. are living with HIV or AIDS. About a quarter of them don't even know they have it.

An HIV-positive woman can also infect her child with HIV before or during childbirth or through breastfeeding. But because this can be prevented with medication, it has become rare in the U.S. (Only 142 children were infected by their mothers in 2005.)

Anyone who has anal sex, male or female, has a high risk of getting infected, because rectal tissues are delicate and can tear easily during sex. Vaginal tissue is also really delicate, so girls who have vaginal sex also have a high risk of getting infected. If you already have another sexually transmitted infection (such as gonorrhea or chlyamidia), you're more likely to get HIV if you're exposed to it.

In general, minority teens, especially African-Americans, are at a high risk: more than half of all youth (13-24) diagnosed with HIV/AIDS in 2004 were African-American even though they are less than 15% of the population. The total number of young people living with AIDS increased by 42% from 2000 to 2004.

What HIV Does To Your Body

Your immune system protects you from getting sick. Your body is exposed to bacteria and other infections each and every second. They would make you ill if you didn't have your immune system, which attacks these invaders by sending white blood cells to destroy them.

HIV goes after the immune system, destroying your white blood cells and leaving your body open to infection and diseases. HIV eventually weakens your immune system so much that you are vulnerable to lots of major health problems, like fever, pneumonia (fluid in the lungs), weight loss, some cancers, and damage to the nervous system (the brain and nerves).

The Symptoms of HIV and AIDS

We can't tell by looking at somebody if that person has HIV because in most cases the infected person doesn't have any visible symptoms. Some people can have HIV for years without getting sick at all. The only way to find out if they have HIV is to get tested.

Other HIV-positive people might start having symptoms like feeling tired often, running a high fever, or losing weight.

The most visible sign of HIV is the lesion: a spot on someone's face, arms, or legs that's red or purple on white skin and bluish, brownish, or black on brown skin.

When the immune system collapses and medication is unable to get rid of HIV symptoms, the person has AIDS. Eventually, your body won't be able to fight back, and you'll die.

Treatment for HIV and AIDS

Today, unlike when HIV first started spreading, we have

drugs that can keep HIV from developing into AIDS. These drugs can't destroy the virus, but they can keep it from copying itself. We also have drugs that strengthen an HIV-positive person's immune system so that it can fight more infections.

Unfortunately, the drugs don't work for everyone. Plus, if they do work at first, the virus can change and find a new way to reproduce. If that happens, the drugs the HIV-positive person is taking won't help anymore, and he has to try a new combination of medicines to keep HIV from attacking his immune system.

Once you start treatment, you may need to continue taking it for the rest of your life. Sometimes a particular treatment combination can work for years and then suddenly stop working. That usually means the virus has developed resistance to the drugs. Sometimes the person develops serious side effects to the drugs and can't take them anymore. When this happens, the doctor will change your medications, if another is available.

If a person starts to show signs of AIDS, the doctor can prescribe drugs to slow down the symptoms and help the patient live longer.

Side Effects of HIV/AIDS Treatment

HIV drugs can keep people alive, but they may cause other problems in the body, called side effects. An HIV-positive person's pills might cause tiredness, stomach pain, fever, insomnia (trouble sleeping), headaches, vomiting, hallucinations, nightmares, or diarrhea.

Medication cannot prevent HIV transmission—you can still infect others even while receiving treatment.

Zaineb was 16 when she wrote this story.

How to Prevent HIV

Since there's no cure for HIV, prevention is key. Abstinence—not having sex—is the only 100% sure way to avoid HIV (plus other STDs and pregnancy). But if you do have sex, here's how to protect yourself:

Get tested, and ask your sexual partner to get tested. Go to www.hivtest.org to find a testing site near you.

Talk to your sex partners about their sexual history and yours. Ask them if they've been tested for HIV, and don't have sex with someone who doesn't know her or his status, even if they seem healthy.

Use condoms. Using condoms during sex can drastically reduce your chances of getting HIV. Even if you and your partner have both been tested for HIV and other STDs, you should use condoms every time you have sex—vaginal, anal, or oral. (Why? See the stories on pp. 38, 41, 44, and 54—even a partner you've been with for many years could be hiding something from you. And keep in mind that condoms are not a foolproof method—they can break.

Don't share needles. If you inject drugs, don't share a needle with anyone else.

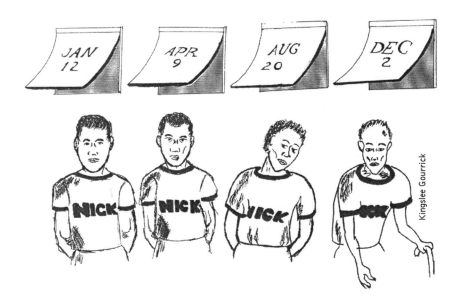

Kingslee Gourrick

Saying Goodbye to Uncle Nick

By Josbeth Lebron

Nick was my stepfather's brother, but I felt more comfortable with him than with my own stepfather. I met him when I was 7 years old, and by the second time I saw him I was already calling him Uncle Nick.

It was just his way of being that I liked: he was honest, sweet, funny, and very understanding. He was the type of person who, the minute you met him, was immediately trying to make you laugh. He did everything he could to make you feel comfortable, and it worked.

I used to see him at least three times a month (which was a lot considering he lived in the Bronx and we live in Queens). We didn't go out much but we always spent time together at my grandmother's house.

Every time I saw him I said, "Hi, Uncle Nick," and he always responded, "What's up, sweetheart, how you doing?" He always asked me how I was doing in school and if I had a boyfriend. When it came to school, I never disappointed him since I always had good grades.

When it came down to boys, I always responded, "No, I don't have a boyfriend," and he would say, "Good, you're too young for boys anyway." He always had new jokes and new ways to make me laugh. Uncle Nick was an all around nice guy. I loved and cared about him very much.

Six years ago, I heard the news that Uncle Nick had the AIDS virus. He was 27 and I was 12. My mother and step-father sat my two step-brothers and me down and explained the whole situation. I was shocked. I couldn't understand how a disease I had just heard of two years before could already be affecting my family. Uncle Nick was such a cool guy; why was this happening to him?

My parents told me and my brothers that we shouldn't act or treat Nick differently, but I already knew that; I wasn't going to treat him like an outcast just because he was sick. But I did expect his illness to show. The surprising thing was that the next time I saw him, he looked fine to me. I guess I expected him to look instantly like a monster, but he looked exactly the same as before.

I thought that maybe he wasn't sick after all. Maybe they had made a mistake—mixed up the blood samples at the laboratory or something like that. Or maybe his immune system was fighting it off and he was going to be OK. I kept all of these thoughts in my mind so I wouldn't have to believe that Uncle Nick had AIDS. This worked for a while but not for too long.

After about a year I began noticing changes in my uncle. They weren't drastic changes, but they were noticeable. At first he gained some weight but he lost it quickly. Then his hair started thinning, which was obvious because he had always had a full head of hair.

About a year and a half after his illness started to show, his wife died. She had AIDS, too. Before they got sick, they had been separated for a while and both of them got involved with other people. That was the origin of their tragedy, I think.

I didn't know Nick's wife that well, so her death did not affect me. But after that, Nick had less hope because he was on his own, trying to fight the battle by himself.

About a month after his wife died, Nick stopped taking his medication. I guess his reasoning was, "What's the point of medication if I'm going to die anyway?" Uncle Nick had lost his hope for living. But his family still had hope and they convinced him to start taking it again. "What a relief," I thought, because to me, his not taking his medication would be like committing suicide.

Seeing someone die of AIDS is like watching a person's life going by on fast-forward.

It was around this time that the physical changes in Uncle Nick became drastic. He must have lost about 30 pounds all at once. It was very noticeable because he was about 6'1" and was down to the bone. He looked skinnier than I do and I only weigh 93 lbs.

He wasn't bald, but his hair was so thin you could see his scalp from a distance. He started getting lesions (they're like sores) on his scalp and on his neck. He began losing his vision and having dizzy spells.

Since the changes were so drastic, they put a certain fear in our hearts which no one spoke of but everyone shared. The fear was that at any moment Uncle Nick could be gone. Seeing someone die of AIDS is like watching a person's life going by on fast-forward. Their aging process hits full speed, and there is no way back. The hair goes. They walk and talk slower. Their face wrinkles and their vision blurs. By the time my uncle was 30, he looked as old as 50.

At night I cried and begged God to let Nick be cured. Every time I listened to the news, I knew there was still hope. There was always new medication out there, and in my heart I always felt there was a chance that Uncle Nick would survive this and that one day we could all laugh about how scared we had been.

Since I first found out he had AIDS, I always kissed Uncle Nick on the cheek. I didn't think anything of it since I knew it wasn't possible to contract his disease in that manner. But when he started getting those lesions, I became scared for myself. I worried that I could catch some kind of infection from him, but I kissed him anyway.

One day Uncle Nick decided he wanted to treat my mother and me to some ice cream. By this time his hands were shaking and he had to walk very slowly. My mother figured he wasn't fit to drive, so she offered to drive his car. I remember him saying, "Nobody's gonna drive that car, only me, that's my car!"

We went and bought the ice cream and we all ordered different flavors. Uncle Nick wanted to taste my ice cream so he grabbed my spoon and took some. Then he joked: "Don't worry, it's not like I have a disease or anything."

I laughed but I was scared because I didn't know if he had any open sores in his mouth, and my gums bleed easily. Even though they say you can't get AIDS from things like that I couldn't help being frightened. So when he wasn't looking, I threw the spoon away and took my mother's.

To this day I still wonder why he did that. But I didn't say anything to him because I didn't want him to feel bad. I didn't want to remind him that he was sick. I wanted him to feel normal.

Uncle Nick fought for his life for as long as he could. I don't think he really believed the virus would kill him. He even seemed to be preparing himself for a new life in the future, as if he had all the time in the world. He bought a new car, rented a new apartment, and bought all new furniture and music equipment. He also got a whole new wardrobe. I felt bad about what he was doing (he was ignoring his illness), but he could afford to buy those things, and since they gave him hope, it was fine with me.

Last June, my mother and I received a phone call from the hospital at one in the morning. Uncle Nick was in the hospital and the doctor said he only had two hours left to live and that we should go see him. My mother went, but I stayed home. I didn't want to see Nick in such pain. I stayed up that night writing poetry in memory of him. Fortunately the doctors were wrong, and my uncle continued to live, but only for two weeks.

While Uncle Nick was in the hospital, his mother slept there to keep him company and to keep an eye on him at all times. Toward the end, while he was still fighting for his life, he would squeeze his mother's hand because he didn't want her to let him go to sleep. I guess he knew he was on his way and he wasn't ready to go. He also didn't want to die in front of anyone. I knew he wanted to die in privacy, because every time my family went to see him in the hospital, he would always say, "Go home, do something, let me rest."

Once he said, "There's a door over there and I don't have the strength to open it, but if you help me I will go." In his dreams he had seen this door and it convinced him that it was time to take a rest. On July 13, Uncle Nick said goodbye to his mother, who was going home for a few hours rest. As he was lying in the hospital room alone, Uncle Nick found the strength to "open the door." I hope that door led him to a new life where there is no pain.

His death didn't hit me hard at first because I couldn't believe he was gone. I saw my mother crying, but I couldn't cry. I said to myself, "Josbeth, what's wrong with you, is your heart made of stone? Your Uncle Nick is dead!" I guess I had to see it to believe it. I thought, "The doctors were wrong before, maybe they're wrong again."

When I went to the funeral parlor I sat in the back of the room but I could still see him from there. Uncle Nick looked like he was sleeping, and I knew he wasn't feeling any pain. I stayed in the back and just cried as I watched my family pay their respects.

I knew he would never awaken from that deep sleep. I didn't want to pay my respects because I wanted to remember him the way he was.

The wake lasted for three days. After the second day I felt guilty because I had never said goodbye to Uncle Nick. I realized this was the last time I would see him, and so I paid my respects. It was really hard for me to say goodbye, but at least I don't feel guilty anymore.

Before this tragedy struck my family I had the feeling that we were invincible. Now I take life a little more seriously.

Before this tragedy struck my family I had the feeling that we were invincible, that nothing could ever harm us. Now I tend to take life a little more seriously. I take into consideration the warnings that are given to me, and I am very cautious about everything, especially sex (I abstain).

I don't think I'll ever forget how serious AIDS is and I want other people to understand that, too. You should never try to fool yourself by thinking, "That can't happen to me," because you're wrong. It could happen to you or to someone you care about. I lost someone very close to me, and the same thing could happen to you. And believe me, it's not easy to lose someone you love.

Josbeth was 17 when she wrote this story. She went on to graduate from high school and go to college.

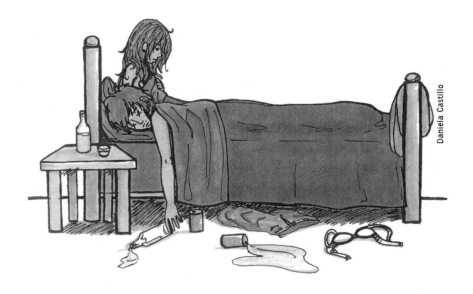

Daniela Castillo

Drunk for One Night, Scared for Six Months

By Anonymous

I had to get tested for HIV/AIDS due to my own stupidity and plain horniness. After a party last spring, I went to my friend's house drunk and had sex without a condom, something my good judgment should have told me not to do.

But my good judgment had disappeared due to the happy, careless feeling that came with the liquor.

As soon as I sobered up, I realized I might have exposed myself to a deadly disease, and I was furious with myself. I'd risked my life. I swore I'd never have unprotected sex again.

On the plus side (if there can be a plus side to playing with death), I hadn't had sex with some random guy. He was one of my closest friends, so I knew I wouldn't feel uncomfortable asking him about his sexual history. His business became my business once we had sex.

I knew that he was far from a virgin, often calling himself a "male whore." But I was stunned when he had to make a list to figure out how many girls he'd slept with. All I could think was, "That is just full out nasty." Yep, I was getting tested for every disease known to man and woman.

Most of the sexually transmitted diseases didn't have me shook—it was HIV that concerned me. I went on the Internet to see how long it takes for HIV to show up in your bloodstream and learned that sometimes it can take up to six months.

I didn't want to feel like I needed to take a test every other day, so I decided to wait the full six months before getting tested.

As soon as I sobered up, I realized I might have exposed myself to a deadly disease, and I was furious with myself.

Then laziness set in. I sort of forgot that I planned on being tested. I became consumed with work and school. However, I made a decision not to have sex again until I was certain that I was free and clear of any diseases. It wouldn't be fair to have sex with someone and unknowingly infect him.

I got tested for every STD other than HIV/AIDS when I went in for my OB-GYN appointment, and I was fine. Then, when World AIDS Day came around in December, I remembered that I wanted to get tested for HIV.

I knew what I had to do and called a youth center to make an appointment to be tested for HIV. It was convenient—I could get tested during my lunch break or on a Saturday.

Before the nurse administered the test, a counselor asked me a bunch of questions. What would I do if I found out that I had HIV? How would I act toward the person who I believed gave me the disease? What would my family and friends say or do if I told them?

After the counselor prepared me for either a negative or positive result, the nurse drew my blood and the test went off to the lab.

I wasn't scared. There was really nothing I could do if I did test positive. I couldn't rewind the hands of time. I would have to accept it, deal with it, and make the best of my life.

I tried to go about the next two weeks without feeling jittery and nervous.

I went back to the youth center two weeks later because that's when my nurse said that the result would be ready. Just my luck, it was late. The nurse promised to mail me a blank postcard when the result came in. I saw myself cursing her out, but I happened to like her and it wasn't her fault.

Waiting those few extra days was worse than the whole six months I'd spent putting off getting tested. I just wanted to know one way or the other.

What would I do if I found out that I had HIV?

Finally the day came when I could go back for my test result. They couldn't tell me over the phone.

After waiting God knows how many hours in the waiting room, the nurse called me in. She told me that I was negative. I didn't need to retest because I hadn't had sex since that night last spring.

The news was terrific and I was beyond excited. But I also remembered what I promised myself after the night's events. After putting myself through all that waiting, I will never be so dumb as to have unprotected sex again, tipsy or otherwise.

The author was 21 when she wrote this story. She graduated from the University of Virginia and went to law school.

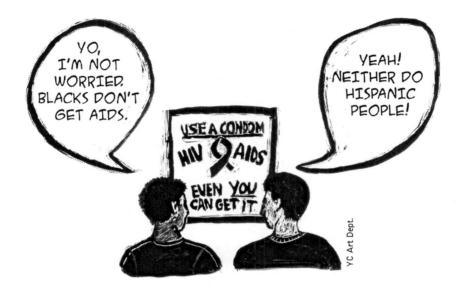

Why Are We Still Taking Risks?

By Orubba Almansouri

Patricia Dittus works at the Centers for Disease Control and Prevention, the nation's public health agency. She studies how teens behave when it comes to protecting ourselves from STDs, and develops ways to help teens, parents, schools and health care providers reduce risky sexual behaviors among adolescents.

I talked to her about why teens keep putting themselves at risk.

Q: It seems some teens who understand how to protect themselves against STDs still engage in risky behaviors. Why might this be?

A: Behavior is really complex. Teens might know that having unprotected sex puts them at risk for STDs, but they might still find themselves in situations in which they're likely to engage in that behavior anyway. Teens need more than just information; they need to be taught important skills that will help protect them—things like refusal skills, negotiation skills, and the skills to seek health care on their own.

They also need to have opportunities to practice those skills. There are role-playing activities in which students can learn about the skill, and then have a chance to practice the skill within the context of a program. Research shows that those kinds of programs show better behavior change later.

Q: What things affect teens' behavior when it comes to protecting themselves against STDs?

A: There are familial influences, like positive relationships with parents and good communication. There are peer influences, like what your friends and classmates consider acceptable behavior. There are school influences, like how connected teens feel to their school, or how much they think teachers care about them, as well as school programs and policies—things like condom availability programs, education programs, after-school activities.

Teens need more than just information; they need to be taught important skills that will help protect them

And there are cultural and societal attitudes about sexuality—for example, the ways American media portray sexuality in ads has an impact on how teens think about their own sexuality, and then might impact how they choose to behave.

Q: What should parents, educators, and lawmakers do to help curb rates of HIV and other STDs among teens?

A: Teens need to be provided with information and skills about the range of prevention and risk-reduction options that are available to them. They also need to know more about how to make good decisions in their lives in general, and they need access to health care services.

Parents, educators and legislators each have a role to play in making sure that teens get these things. For example, parents can talk to their teens about sex in terms of how to weigh the consequences, how to make decisions about sex. Parents can keep track of their teens and make sure they set limits on their behavior, especially behaviors that might contribute to risk—like dating somebody older, or getting involved in drugs.

Orubba was 16 when she conducted this interview.

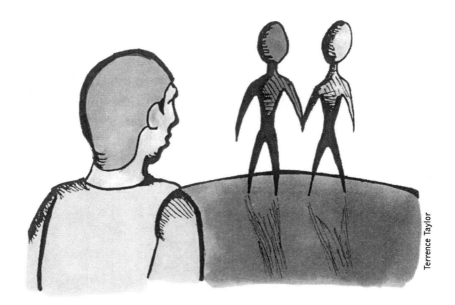

Terrence Taylor

Keeping Quiet

By Anonymous

How would you define a friend? For me, a friend is someone you know well and who knows you well, someone with whom you share affection and respect. Along with friendship comes a degree of responsibility to support each other in a time of need or crisis. But how far does that responsibility go?

I met KaJuan last summer through one of my other friends. We clicked right away and hung out every day, all summer. We went to the beach and hung out at gay nightclubs. Since I'm an excellent dancer, I tried to teach him different dance moves. It was funny to see him struggling to learn the moves.

I found him attractive and thought we would make a great couple. But we talked about it and agreed that a relationship wouldn't last as long as a friendship. We decided not to risk our friendship and, three weeks later, KaJuan started dating another guy.

I felt fine about that until recently, when my friend Robert gave me some shocking news about KaJuan's new boyfriend. Robert said that he used to go out with KaJuan's boyfriend. Since Robert is HIV-positive, he only dates men who are HIV-positive as well. That's how he knew that KaJuan's boyfriend has had HIV for five years. Robert wanted me to keep this a secret because no one else knew about his own HIV status.

I didn't want to believe what I had just heard. KaJuan had previously told me that he and his new boyfriend have had unprotected sex numerous times. He said it was OK because they were in a committed relationship and knew each other's HIV status was negative. Or so he thought.

I felt like a rag doll being pulled apart by two pre-kindergarten students. I had no idea what to do. Should I tell KaJuan about his boyfriend's HIV status or should I keep my mouth shut and avoid getting into drama over someone else's business?

Part of me wanted to tell KaJuan because I care about him and never want to see him hurt. But in the past, I have found myself getting into arguments and have even lost friends because I told other people's personal business, and I was really tired of it. I didn't want KaJuan's boyfriend to accuse me of lying, since it would be his word against mine, and I wasn't sure who KaJuan would believe.

I decided to keep my mouth shut. I felt like I wasn't in a position to reveal KaJuan's boyfriend's personal business, even though I knew it could be a matter of life or death. I also felt that KaJuan shouldn't have believed his boyfriend's status just based on what his boyfriend said. When KaJuan got tested, he showed his boyfriend his actual results from the clinic. He should have asked his boyfriend to do the same thing.

It has been two months since I found out and, as far as I know, KaJuan still does not know that his boyfriend has HIV. I feel so guilty that I haven't opened my mouth. I really hope that

KaJuan doesn't contract HIV. If he does, I would feel devastated because he would be the second person I know with the disease. I would also feel somewhat responsible for not telling him.

I try to make up for not telling KaJuan by promoting safe sex to him. I often point out the risk of having unprotected sex and the consequences, reminding him that it's not just HIV he has to watch out for, but many other STDs. I think KaJuan listens to what I have to say, because he often says stuff like, "For real? I didn't know that."

Should I tell KaJuan about his boyfriend's HIV status or should I keep my mouth shut?

I still feel strongly that it's not my place to reveal KaJuan's boyfriend's status. That's his boyfriend's responsibility. The only thing that I feel I can do is try to convince KaJuan to start practicing safe sex. But sometimes I still feel like I'm not being a friend to KaJuan because I'm holding out on information that could change his life forever.

The author was 18 when he wrote this story.

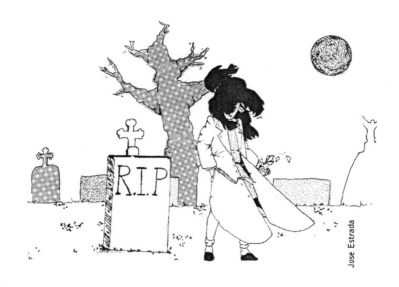

Jose Estrada

My Uncle Died of Aids...
And I Still Love Him

By Anonymous

My uncle died of AIDS. It's hard to admit and hard to talk about. When my family finally admitted it was AIDS, it was too late—he was dead.

Jay was married, but he also had sex with other men. His wife, Renee, never knew he had sex with other men until after 10 years of marriage. At times, Uncle Jay would tell his wife he was going out for a night of fun with the guys. Little did she know how he meant it.

When relatives or friends dropped by unexpectedly and he was "entertaining," it was a bit awkward. From what I saw, no one acknowledged his sexual activity. It was OK as long as nobody talked about it at Grandma's Thanksgiving dinner.

The first time I heard that Jay was in the hospital, I never even thought it might be AIDS—it never entered my mind. My aunt Liza was frightened because the doctors asked her whether he had ever been an intravenous drug user. Soon, other close family members received phone calls from the doctors, and the paranoia began.

When Liza questioned the doctors, they told her they suspected he had been exposed to the HIV virus. She fell apart at the seams. How do you tell other family members that a loved one is dying? Renee told us that Uncle Jay had specifically asked that no one be told.

As I think back on it, Jay's death was a tragic one. He was all alone, except for his wife and the nurses who began to know him by name. My cousin asked me to go see him, but I claimed I was too busy. I wasn't too busy to go, but too scared. Now I realize that was the biggest cop-out I've ever had a part in.

From what I was told, Jay really needed someone to talk to, just a new face. He was trying to hang on to what little dignity he had left. His health had deteriorated quickly, and he died within a year of being tested.

Jay was very special to all of us, but somehow my family wasn't able to admit he was dying.

Jay was very special to all of us, but somehow my family wasn't able to admit he was dying. It became very clear to me that homosexuality is still a taboo subject in America. Only three people were at Jay's funeral. I didn't go because I wanted to say goodbye on my own.

One Saturday I went to the cemetery. I told him I loved him and would try not to discriminate against people who had chosen a different route. I'm angry at Uncle Jay, my family, and myself for not being able to accept him for what he was. Nobody should stop loving someone because of their sexual orientation, or because they have AIDS.

Please, if you know someone who is afflicted, don't let them suffer alone. After they're gone, you can't make it up to them. Goodbye, Uncle Jay. I still love you.

The author was in high school when she wrote this story.

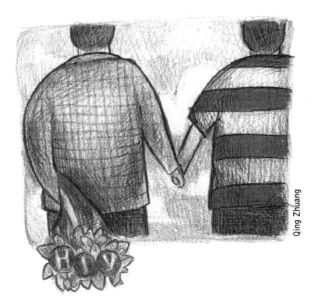

Date With Destiny

By Anonymous

Let me tell you about the day that changed my destiny. It was July 30, 1998. Ten days after I turned 20 years old. I had a job at a health center in New York, and I was excited about getting my own place soon.

Two weeks before, I had gotten tested for HIV. I started getting tested when I was 16 years old because I was having sex and sometimes didn't use a condom.

I had always gotten a negative result, meaning I didn't have HIV. And since the last time I'd been tested, the only person I'd had unprotected sex with was my long-term boyfriend. He assured me that he had been tested for HIV and that he did not have it. He refused to show me the test results, but I trusted him. He had been asking me to have unprotected sex for some time, and I eventually gave in. The condoms went out the window for the duration of our relationship.

After about a year and a half, our relationship ended. It wasn't long before I was over him and loving being single.

So back to July 30. When it was time to go see what my results were, I said a prayer. In the waiting room, I thumbed through a magazine but I couldn't read any of the articles. I always felt a little anxiety waiting for the results of my HIV test.

"Excuse me, Pedro?" a voice called out, interrupting my thoughts.

"Let's go into my office so we can have a little more privacy," the HIV counselor said.

She told me what the three possible test results were, the stuff you hear every time you get tested for HIV. It was either: negative, meaning I didn't have HIV; inconclusive, meaning the test was unable tell whether I had HIV and I would need to be tested again; or positive, meaning I had contracted HIV.

As she went on, I got more and more anxious. I really just wanted to know what the results were.

I had trusted my ex, and he had failed me. I felt like he took my life away from me.

Then she told me what I would need to do if I was negative. "Be sure to continue practicing safe sex, get tested in six months, and be with only one partner," she said, sounding like a mother telling me to wear clean socks.

I tuned her out then because I didn't want to think about it.

"OK, and now for your results," she said.

"Ladies and gentlemen, the envelope please," I thought to myself.

She opened the file and placed it on her desk.

"Pedro, your results came back positive," she blurted.

The blood ran from my body. I was in shock. How? Why? But most of all, who? Who gave me HIV?

I swallowed and tried to compose myself. I kept telling myself to breathe. Why me? I was so young.

I felt as if I had let down people who cared about me. I felt guilty for being gay. I felt like this was a punishment from God. I did everything possible to prevent myself from crying.

"Are you OK?" she was asking.

"Yeah, fine." It was a lie, of course.

"You might want to take a few days off to relax and absorb this. This is not going to be easy for you, but you can do it. Understand that this does not mean a death sentence."

Everything else she said was just a blur. I couldn't listen anymore. I needed to leave. I wanted to go home and crawl into bed. I didn't want to think about this. Not now.

I went straight to my boss's office. I told her that I needed to leave immediately. She allowed me to take off the next two days. I went outside and walked around aimlessly for two hours.

I was angry, so angry. I didn't know what to do with myself so I decided to go see my ex to tell him what had happened. I was confident that he was the one who infected me.

By the time I got to his house, I was fuming mad. I wanted answers and I wanted them yesterday.

"How could you do this to me?" I asked.

"Who did you tell?" he wanted to know. He didn't want any of my friends getting revenge on him.

"What does it matter? I told those who are concerned about me."

"You shouldn't have done that. Why didn't you call me first? We could have handled this together."

"No, we couldn't have," I replied, getting more agitated by the moment. "Look, all I want to know is, are you positive?"

"Uh, yeah, I just got tested recently and I found out I'm positive."

"You what?" My voice was getting louder and I was beginning to get choked up. I couldn't believe this was happening. "I think you've been positive longer than you say you have. How could you do this? I asked you over and over if you were negative and you lied to me! What am I supposed to do now?"

"Listen, baby, we can work this out." He tried to pull me closer to him.

"Get off of me! There is nothing to work out!" I pulled away from him. I had heard enough. "F-ck you! Don't ever bother me again!" I screamed. I was crying now. There was nothing more to say or do. I picked up my book bag, wiped my face with my shirt and stormed out of his house. My head was pounding. I could hear him calling me to come back. I kept walking.

I went home and got in bed. I felt as if my life had stopped. I had so many emotions swirling in my head that I could not even think straight.

As I lay in my bed, I remembered all the people I already knew who were living with HIV.

I promised myself that I would not give up without a fight.

They were able to do everything they wanted to do in their lives. Nothing stopped them. Their sense of humor about it also helped them to deal with it better. Remembering them made me feel a little calmer.

I knew I could talk to them about what I was going through. I also knew I had many other people who could help support me. I kept telling myself that I was fortunate to have tested positive in 1998 and not 1988, a time when little was known about HIV and there were very few medications available.

But I was also pissed off. Although the responsibility of deciding to have unsafe sex fell in my lap, I was angry because I had given my ex the benefit of the doubt. I had trusted him. And he had failed me. I felt like he took my life away from me.

I wanted to get even with him for lying to me. But deep inside, I knew that revenge would get me nowhere. Afterward, I would still be HIV-positive. Nothing could change that.

I fell asleep hoping that when I awoke, this day would have been a dream.

After several weeks, once the initial shock wore off, I began looking for ways that I could improve my life, both physically and emotionally. I'd never allowed any challenge in my life to take me down before and I was not about to let this one be the first.

I began to go to therapy to help myself deal with being HIV-positive. Therapy taught me that although I may be faced with a life-threatening illness, I shouldn't use it as a reason for not trying to achieve the things I want in life. In fact, it should be the reason for achieving the goals I want, such as finishing college. I promised myself that I would not give up without a fight.

I started spending a lot of time alone, just looking at my life. If I wanted to live longer, I knew that I needed to spend more time on me and less time in the clubs. I needed to make sure that I got enough rest, reduced my stress, and took my medications.

Above all, though, I needed to practice safe sex at all times. I did not want to infect another person. I did not want to live the rest of my days knowing that I was responsible for that.

I went back to college soon after finding out that I was HIV-positive. I wrote a final report, which was close to 175 pages, about learning to cope with HIV. Writing really helped me put what happened to me over the past year into perspective. It helped me realize how strong a person I really was. It also helped me find ways of coping, such as exercising, talking more with my friends, and taking acupuncture when life was getting too stressful for me.

I got an A+ on the paper and was the only student in my class to make it onto the dean's list that semester.

This past summer marked three years since I learned that I was positive. I am now working as the administrative director for a community foundation, and am still trying to finish that college degree.

My viral load is undetectable, which means that the amount of HIV in my body is so low that the current available tests cannot detect it. It does not mean that I am negative, it just means that there isn't a lot of HIV in my system. This is due, in part, to me taking my medications and living a healthier life.

More important, I have gradually managed to come to terms with my HIV status. I've learned to forgive myself for being HIV-positive. I don't consider this a punishment from God. I consider it sort of like a tap on the shoulder telling me that I need to take better care of myself and not be so reckless with my life.

Believe it or not, I also forgave the person who infected me. I had the opportunity to protect myself and I chose not to. I can live with that. Being angry at him or trying to be vengeful towards him will not make the HIV leave my body. I want to live a happy life, not a bitter one. Although he is no longer in my life, I know that I would be able to see him in the street and not want to get into a fistfight with him.

> **Being angry at my ex will not make the HIV leave my body. I want to live a happy life, not a bitter one.**

Now that I'm living with HIV I have learned to be grateful for what I have. The expensive medications I need are covered by my health insurance. There are so many in this world who don't even know they have HIV, or don't have access to the costly care they need.

I am looking forward to living a healthy, long life. My doctor tells me that if I take my medications and follow his orders, he can help me live to the age of 60. And with all the research going on about HIV, maybe, just maybe, they might come up with a cure.

The author was 24 when he wrote this story. He graduated from college and went on to work at a major media company.

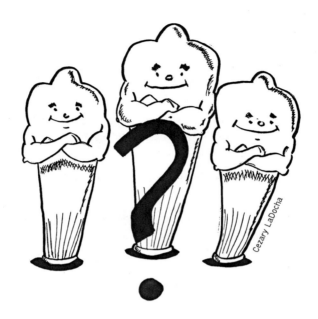

Cezary LaDocha

How Reliable Are Condoms?

By Ashley Amey

A few weeks ago, I was reading a book by Hasani Pettiford, a motivational speaker. My mother told me to read it because she wanted me to get better educated about sex and doing right by God.

Pettiford's a Christian who believes that life would be much easier if people just waited until they're married to have sex, and that having sex any time before marriage is sinful.

The topic that stood out the most to me in his book was "Condoms (How Safe Are They?)" This surprised me because I'd never seen a writer question how reliable condoms are. Pettiford referred to several doctors who said that people shouldn't rely on condoms as a form of protection against sexually transmitted infections.

I doubted that this man knew what he was talking about,

because he wasn't a health professional. I thought this book might be trying to discourage readers from having sex outside of marriage by trying to exaggerate the risks associated with using a condom.

I wanted to find out if what he claimed was true, so I began to do research. Most of what I found showed that Pettiford's "facts" weren't true.

I visited the website of the Centers for Disease Control (CDC), the top government agency committed to providing reliable health information to the public.

The CDC published a 1993 report on how well condoms protect against HIV infection and other sexually transmitted diseases. The report shows that a properly used latex condom provides a high degree of protection against different sexually transmitted infections, including HIV.

The CDC said other studies show that 98-100% of people who use condoms correctly and consistently did not become infected if they were sexually involved with people who had HIV. The organization made clear that when engaging in sexual intercourse, you can greatly reduce your risk of getting (or giving) sexually transmitted infections by using a condom.

A properly used latex condom provides a high degree of protection against different sexually transmitted infections, including HIV.

Then I contacted three health professionals. They all felt that condoms were the most effective way to have safer anal, oral, or vaginal sex.

"Condoms are not perfect, but if they are used consistently and correctly, they are very helpful," said Dr. David Rose, who's the former director of the AIDS center at Mount Sinai Hospital. "They are a good way of protecting oneself from many STDs, such as gonorrhea, syphilis, and hepatitis B, as well as HIV."

Maggie Janes, a health coordinator and HIV counselor for Mount Sinai Adolescent Health Care Center, agreed that condoms are highly effective in protecting against HIV, since HIV can be transmitted through oral, anal, or vaginal sex. She also said that condoms are 95%–97% effective in preventing pregnancy when used correctly.

I asked Janes what she thought about Pettiford's statements that condoms aren't safe. Janes disagreed, and referred to tests done by the U.S. Food and Drug Administration which allows no more than 4 out 1,000 condoms to leak during random checks of condom samples taken from warehouses.

*J*anes said abstinence is the only sure way to avoid pregnancy or STDs, but that when you use condoms correctly each time you have sex, you are drastically decreasing your chances of getting infected or getting pregnant.

Studies show that condoms are more effective against certain infections than others, and it's best to consult with health professionals to find out the level of protection a condom can give you against certain diseases.

Some health officials also say that studies on condom effectiveness show varying rates because some studies measure typical use. Typical use refers to when people use condoms both correctly and incorrectly; studies that include incorrect use of a condom will show a higher rate of condom failure than studies that measure the perfect use of a condom.

Condoms can tear or slip off if they're not being used correctly. Being drunk or high increases the chance that you'll make a mistake.

Officials recommend that if you're not used to using a condom, you should carefully follow the directions on the wrapping; guys should practice putting the condom on and off and masturbating with it on to get used to the sensation.

Users should take into account condom strength, sensitivity, size, and lubrication, depending on the type of sex they're having; for instance, anal sex is thought to put more strain on a condom than vaginal sex.

According to Nora Gelperin, a training coordinator for The Network for Family Life Education at Rutgers University in New Jersey, latex condoms work best when they're used with spermicides like nonoxynol-9, which helps kill sperm. (Many condoms come with spermicide already on them.) Gelperin advises always using both condoms and another type of contraception, like the pill.

"Teens can take precautions by talking to their partners, going to the doctor for annual check-ups, talking to doctors, using more than one source of protection (condoms, the pill, or Depo-Provera), and sharing their history with their current partner," Janes said.

After completing my research and interviews, I don't feel like condoms are perfect, but they greatly reduce the chances of getting an STD or becoming pregnant. If you're going to have sex, condoms are the best way to protect yourself from STDs, including HIV. I see condoms as a way of practicing "safer," not "safe" sex, since it's only abstinence that lowers the risks associated with sex to zero.

Ashley was 16 when she wrote this story. She graduated from high school and went to Virginia State University.

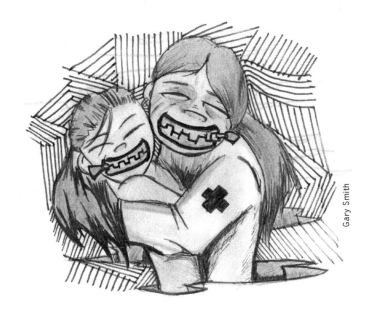

Gary Smith

A Sad Silence

By Desirée Guéry

There was a secret in my family that went on for years. Well, it wasn't a secret to everyone, only to me. One day, on a drive home with my dad, he told me, "Your Aunt Sheila is sick."

Aunt Sheila was my father's sister, my Titi. We were close and spoke on the phone about every two weeks. I thought it was strange that she didn't tell me herself that she was sick.

"Sick?" I asked curiously. "With the flu?"

"No, she has AIDS," he said blankly, staring at the scenery outside. He said it as if it were no big deal, as if it wouldn't affect me.

Being only 8 or 9, I didn't understand what AIDS was. I had no idea it's a deadly disease. I just nodded, thinking nothing of it. My father didn't make a big deal of it, and they were close, so I figured it must not be serious and felt no need to continue the conversation. I had no idea how devastated I'd feel later on.

My mother, who I was closer to, talked to me more about it later that night. Titi Sheila had wanted to keep her illness a secret from me so that she could find a way to tell me herself. Mom said she caught the disease from someone she loved and trusted—her fiancé.

I didn't understand what she meant when she said Titi got the disease from her partner, but I didn't ask any questions since Mom said I wasn't supposed to know. Maybe Mom didn't want to tell me much so that the news would still be somewhat fresh when Titi told me.

But Titi didn't bring it up.

I saw her a few times after my talk with my parents during her yearly visits from Montreal, Canada, where she lived. She looked as I always remembered her: healthy.

She had meat on her bones and looked vivacious and gorgeous in clothes she made herself. She was a fashion designer, and was often decked out with embroidered scarves, makeup, and gold jewelry.

I always looked forward to her visits and our trips shopping together, when she'd buy scarves and purses. She was free-spirited, fun, fashionable, and loving, which is what I remember most about her.

I didn't know how to bring up Titi's illness when I was with her, so I didn't. But I began to better understand what she had when I learned about AIDS in 6th and 7th grades.

I soon realized that AIDS was a condition that developed from being infected with HIV, a virus you get through unprotected sex or sharing needles. Because of the AIDS virus, her immune system had shut down.

Because her immune system wasn't working, it was harder, if not impossible, for her to fight off other viruses, such as a cold or the flu. Catching those viruses could lead to bigger illnesses as well.

It was frightening learning about a disease that hit so close to home while my classmates seemed like they couldn't care less about the topic. I couldn't keep my emotions bottled up. I often cried in class. One of my best friends at the time, Jackie, would console me. I'd told her about Titi Sheila's condition. I trusted her and needed someone to talk to about how I was feeling.

It was nice to have a shoulder to cry on and a friend to talk to who knew just as much about the disease as I did. But I didn't talk to Mom about it. After learning about AIDS, and hearing comments all day on the subject, I didn't want to go home and discuss it any further.

Still, I feel horrible about never hearing the words come straight from Titi Sheila's mouth about her condition. I think I would've understood her illness more if we'd discussed it. I wanted her to tell me how she felt. I hate not knowing how she felt then, and I hate knowing that she'll never be able to tell me.

She probably wasn't comfortable discussing it with me, even though when we talked, I told her whatever was on my mind. I wish she'd done the same. At times, I felt like she didn't trust me, or thought I couldn't handle her condition.

Maybe I never gave her the opportunity to talk to me about her illness since I was often so busy talking about a celebrity crush I had or something that happened in school. But I figured that if she didn't want to tell me about her illness, I shouldn't ask.

But the changes I soon noticed spoke mountains. When I was 13, Titi Sheila visited us. Her physical appearance had changed dramatically. Although her personality was still lively and bubbly, she was stick thin.

I'd never seen her that thin before. I was scared for her. I knew she must be really sick. I remember her showing my mother and me how she had to wear extra clothes and "butt pads" under her jeans to make them fit.

Even with all the extra layers and padding, she was the thinnest person I'd ever seen. I overheard her telling my mother she'd lost her appetite.

"I can barely keep anything down," she said. I understood much more about the disease at this point, but didn't know that AIDS could cause you to lose your appetite and weight.

She was always catching small colds, the sniffles, stomach-aches, and headaches. Even though these are normal things people catch, for Titi, it was bad. Her immune system was shut down, so a simple cold could turn into pneumonia. Titi often had to go to the hospital. I felt terrible that she had to have it worse than most.

Titi Sheila still wouldn't tell me about her illness, even though she must've known I

Her immune system was shut down, so a simple cold could turn into pneumonia.

could see how poor her health was. Plus I'd overhear my mother talking to her, or see my mother crying because Titi was in the hospital or home in bed for weeks. I worried, but whenever I spoke to Titi and asked how she was feeling, she assured me she was doing fine.

But three years ago, in August, she took a trip to Spain with her boyfriend and caught a small stomach flu. "I was at the hotel for most of the trip," she told me when she got home. "I just kept throwing up. It's just a small stomach bug. It'll go away."

It didn't. She was admitted to the hospital a week after arriving home.

My parents and I visited her in the hospital in Montreal. To see her so sick, barely able to do anything herself, not even able to stay awake, hurt me more than any physical pain I'd experienced. I cried all day, and it was hard, because I didn't want her to see me cry.

I knew it might be the last time I'd ever see her since she was so sick. I couldn't handle the thought of growing up without her humor, love, guidance, understanding, and support.

I wanted so badly to tell her that I knew, since I knew I'd probably never have the chance to talk to her about it again. But I just couldn't. I didn't know how to say it, or how she'd react, so

I brought up other things.

A few weeks after we got back home, my grandmother, who was still with Titi at the hospital, told my mother and me that Titi was feeling better. We were relieved.

Then, about two weeks after Grandma said Titi was doing better, the phone rang at around 2 a.m.

After Mom got off the phone, she started crying. She turned to me and said, "Sheila didn't make it." And we both cried on the couch.

I cried myself to sleep that night. I couldn't believe she'd passed so suddenly when we thought she was getting better.

Mom and I didn't go to her funeral, which was held in Canada, but my father did. Mom said it would be too depressing to go. She didn't want her last vision of Titi to be in a casket.

I felt the same way my mother did. I wanted to remember Titi for what she'd given to me and shown me throughout the years, and that's how I remember her now.

Still, I felt awful. Mom was concerned. "Do you want to talk to me about it?" she asked. "How do you feel?" I just avoided her questions by telling her I wanted to be alone or had nothing to say. She wanted to be there for me, but I wanted to be by myself. Maybe that's how Titi Sheila felt when she was sick.

I never talked to anyone about my feelings over her death, even though it's affected me deeply. I wonder how dealing with Titi's illness would've been different if we'd talked about it.

I think we would've become even closer. But I'll never know, and maybe that's just how she wanted it.

Titi Sheila's death has left me questioning my romantic future. My Titi caught HIV from her fiancé, who'd been cheating on her. I was shocked and disgusted to hear he was having unprotected sex with not just one other woman, but many, and one of them happened to have HIV. Sheila was betrayed by the person whom she thought she could always trust.

Now I feel like I can't completely trust anyone. I'll never

know what goes on behind closed doors. The person I trust with my life could do as Titi's fiancé did, and throw my life away.

My fear of being betrayed is one reason why I haven't dated much. Plus, I'm a picky person. Since I'm reluctant to trust anyone, it's easy for me to find something (or many things) wrong with someone who likes me.

Nowadays, according to Planned Parenthood, about 50% of high school teens report having had sex, even with all the sexually transmitted diseases out there. From stories I've seen and heard, some teens have sex (often unprotected sex) just to have it, and don't think of the consequences.

Titi Sheila's death has left me questioning my romantic future. I feel like I can't completely trust anyone.

I'm planning not to have sex until I'm married. And even though it's pretty much expected for a married couple to have unprotected sex with each other, I don't know if I'll be able to do that.

Just because someone's my husband won't stop me from wondering, "What if he's cheating on me?" or "What if I get a disease?"

I don't think I can have unprotected sex with my future husband until I know for sure that he loves me back and is in love only with me.

The only time I can imagine myself having unprotected sex at this point is if I'm planning on having children, but even the thought of that is a little shaky. What if my aunt was trying to have children? She never had any, and the one person she would've had them with gave her a deadly disease.

Desirée was 16 when she wrote this story.

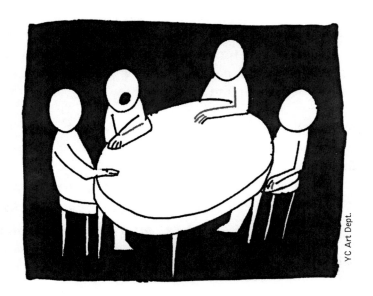

All Too Real:
Teens Living With HIV

Danielle was diagnosed with HIV when she was born in 1989. Doctors gave her three years to live. Sean found out he was HIV-positive last year, and worried at first that he wouldn't live to see his next birthday.

But Danielle and Sean, now 21, are both alive and well, and getting support from Health and Education Alternatives for Teens (HEAT), a community-based program in Brooklyn, New York. The program provides medical and mental health services and case management to youth ages 13-24 who are living with or at high risk for HIV/AIDS.

We talked to them about what it means to live as a young person with the virus today, and what all teens should know about HIV.

Q: How did you contract HIV?

Sean: I was messing with a guy for about a year and a half, and he was married, older. I always used a condom. But this particular night, I was a little drunk, and as I'm having sex with him, I'm realizing that he's not wearing a condom. The back of my mind was telling him to stop, but the words weren't coming out. I told myself, "He's the only guy I've been messing with for the past year, so if I had something, by now I guess it would have shown up."

The back of my mind was telling him to stop, but the words weren't coming out.

Within about five months, I noticed I felt more tired. I got tested, and I was negative. I kept on sleeping with him, and then I stopped, because he was getting on my nerves. Then I went to Job Corps, and they required HIV testing. They told me I was positive.

Through it all, I blame myself. I keep thinking about when we were doing it: the condom was right there. Something in my heart was telling me to stop him, but I was just so caught up in the moment.

Danielle: I got it from my mom—this was before they had drugs to prevent mothers from passing the virus on to their babies. She got it from her husband. (Unlike Danielle, about 80% of HEAT program participants got HIV through sexual activity.)

When my diagnosis came, they told my family that 6 years old was the oldest that I would live to be, and my mom had six more months to live.

With my mom, they actually were right on the money. So I didn't have a chance to go back and ask questions about how or why. My father died a year after my mom, and I didn't know him regardless. So I'm the lone ranger in my family as far as having HIV, with no one to relate to, no one to ask questions.

Q: When did you first discover that you were HIV-positive? What helped you through?

Sean: I discovered I was HIV-positive on March 8, 2008. I was crying, depressed. I didn't go out with friends, because I was scared that I would just walk out the door and drop dead.

My mother died of cancer, and she was living with it for about 18 years. I think the fact that she was fighting just to see her kids grow up reminded me that even though I have HIV, I can't let it beat me. My goal is to live to my 90th birthday. So you could say my mother was my strength.

Danielle: My family found out when I was 3 years old. I was about 7 or 8 when my guardian started seeing me get upset. I said, "Why am I the only one in my class who has to take medicine every day?" She finally sat me down and explained to me that I'm going to be sick, and I could get worse if I don't keep taking my medicine.

Even though I have HIV, I can't let it beat me.

At about 17, I finally understood what HIV was and what it was doing to me. For a while I closed myself off to a lot of people. But I had friends my age who were dealing with the same thing I was dealing with, and that helped pull me through.

Q: How have people reacted when you've told them you're HIV-positive?

Danielle: For years, I never told anybody. In May 2007, they were having a health fair at my church, and they invited a group of my friends from the clinic to come tell their stories. I went up to the podium and words started coming out. After that, I really didn't care. By this time I was 20 and I said, "I'm too old to be holding secrets."

Everybody was cool with it because we were already family. Later I wrote this long email to my high school friends explaining everything. When I clicked "send," I was very nervous.

I got a flood of responses, like, "Oh, my God, you're my she-ro," and, "I can't believe you're so strong…" I loved the support. But honestly, if I'd told them while I was in high school, I don't think it would have been the same.

Q: Do teens know enough about protecting themselves?

Sean: Kids are starting to have sex at 13, and I was one of them. When you're 13, HIV doesn't cross your mind. As you get older, in high school, you think, "OK, he may have HIV—but I highly doubt it, 'cause he's on the basketball team; he looks real good." And you go out there and you take that chance without using a condom.

Danielle: I've seen the curriculum where kids are supposed to learn about HIV. Here's the problem: you can teach through text-books all you want to, but it's not real to them so it doesn't sink in. That's why I don't have a problem telling my status to young people, because that's the only way they're actually going to learn. I tell my story and they see a young face who has it, they start paying attention.

Q: How has HIV impacted your life, including your dating life?

Sean: I've gone on dates. Oral sex, yes, with a condom. Anal sex, no, scared to death.

I told one guy I was messing with that I was HIV-positive, and I spit that out because I was drunk. I was like, "Look, before you get any ideas, I'm HIV-positive." He said, "Oh, that's cool with me." I put a condom on him and just performed oral sex. I wasn't going that far because I was scared the condom might pop and I might be too drunk to notice it.

Honestly, I'm more nervous about what they can give me, because I don't think my body can handle anything else. I'm not trying to catch no STD, or another strain of HIV.

Danielle: I don't even remember that I'm HIV-positive most of the time. Taking my medicine during the day is the only time I remember. Or I might get sick one day and I'm like, "Oh my gosh, I hope it's not because of this."

I'll see somebody at the club and if I see that they like me and I like them, I'll be like, "Hi, my name is so-and-so. I have HIV." Straight up, right after my name. Then I leave it up to them, because I've done my job.

Q: What would you tell teens who are not HIV-positive?

Danielle: I would tell teens, I'm living with this 22 years. I'm 22. And I'm expecting that I will never see a cure.

There is absolutely no escape after getting HIV. Whatever you can do—use a condom, a dental dam, whatever they've got out there. Saran wrap it, I don't care what you've gotta do, use some type of protection.

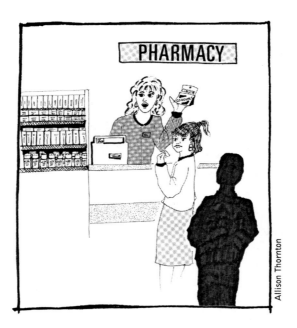

Allison Thornton

Scared to Buy Rubbers?
So Was I!

By Cassaundra Worrell

The big day came. I was going to buy some rubbers—and the only way I felt comfortable about it was to buy them in a different neighborhood. I walked into the supermarket. I laughed to myself and figured no one had spotted me. Little did I know.

Beads of sweat formed across my brow. I waited as the area around the cash register slowly emptied before I approached. In a small voice I asked for the intimidating item.

A slow grin spread across the cashier's face. He then asked in a booming voice, "Lubricated or dry?" When I said "Yes," he realized he had yet another victim. He went for the kill.

By now I was ready to crack, because there was a line of people waiting behind me. With that menacing grin, he screamed, "Ribbed or regular, colored or clear, flavored or without taste, lambskin or latex, edible or non-edible, and what size box?"

By this time I was ready to make in my pants. "Regular, please, and the largest box you have." I added the last part so I would never have to come back.

I got the courage to look him in the face and saw that his name tag said "Mike."

Mike's face got red from laughter as he told me the condoms were kept in the pharmacy department.

Am I the only one who has gone through the trauma of purchasing condoms?

My classmates who will read this may wonder how I managed. "Weren't you afraid that someone would laugh at you?" I certainly was, but I survived, and you can, too.

If you're afraid to buy any form of birth control, you shouldn't be having sex.

Don't you get tired of hearing your parents ask, "When are you going to grow up and accept your responsibilities?" Having safer sex is one of the responsibilities that they're talking about. No matter what your friends may say, you're maturing. If you are thinking about having safer sex, you are a cut above the rest.

If you are already having sex and you are thinking about buying condoms, you deserve a pat on the back—at least you're starting somewhere.

It was so degrading to have "Mike" laugh in my face and to have the people on line behind me look at me with "shame, shame, shame" written across their foreheads.

I know that buying a condom can be rough the first time, but at least you are taking responsibility for your actions, and it could just save your life. Think about this as you ask for that box of condoms—being embarrassed is much better than being dead.

Food for thought: If you're afraid to buy any form of birth

control, you shouldn't be having sex.

Cassaundra was 17 when she wrote this story.
She later went to college and worked as a legal researcher.

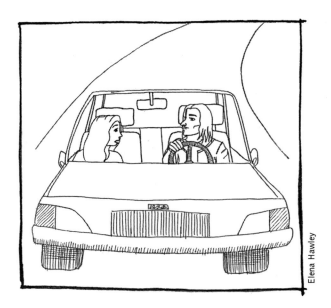

Elena Hawley

My Favorite Uncle Is HIV-Positive

By Kia Thomas

I always knew there was something quite different about my uncle.

When I was little I even wondered how he could be an uncle at all when, to my eyes, he acted and looked just like a woman. My uncle would spend a long time at the mirror doing his hair, plucking his eyebrows, putting different creams on his face, and shaping his lips with lipliner. I even remember asking him why he never wore a skirt like other women.

It wasn't until I was around 6 that I realized that my uncle really was a man. A couple of years later I figured out that one of the things that was different about him was that he liked other men. I would wonder why he and his male friends acted like a man and a woman do—not sexually but just in terms of the closeness that they had with each other.

The fact that my uncle is gay never upset me because in my family it was always accepted. If anything, my uncle's being gay has helped me. Every time I am having guy problems, he's the one I go to for advice because I know he'll understand.

I think I cherish our relationship so much because, out of all my family, my uncle is the only one who understands what it is like to be a teenager. In some ways he is still like a teenager himself. My uncle has a different attitude about life than most adults. Unlike my "boring" parents, he has never settled down. He hangs out with his friends just like I do. He still goes out to clubs and parties till all times of the night.

He also has a crazy sense of humor. If you do something stupid like I tend to do, he makes sure everybody in the family hears about it over and over again. My father is his favorite target. He's the oldest brother and my uncle loves to talk about how old he acts. He is always telling me, "Your father is jealous of me because he's old and bitter and I am young and lovely." In spite of the jokes, their relationship is very close.

He told me there is not a man in the world worth dying for. I agree 100%.

My uncle doesn't just keep me entertained, he also listens to my problems and gives me advice when I need it. For instance, this past summer I was seeing a guy six years older than me and my parents didn't like it. My mother stopped trusting me even though she didn't have a reason to and my father treated me like a child who was unable to have her own life. It was the worst time of my life because it seemed as though my family had turned against me.

The only person I could talk to was my uncle. I told him all about the guy, things I didn't tell anybody else. I asked him if I should continue to see him or call it quits because my family disapproved of our friendship. My uncle told me to do what was best for me because nobody can live my life but Kia. He also said that if I wasn't doing anything wrong then I shouldn't let my parents upset me. I followed his advice and did what I thought was best for me.

When I was 13, I found out something that has changed my life. I was sitting on my grandmother's bed doing nothing when my mother came in the room and told me that she had something to tell me. My curious ears perked up instantly. She looked at me and said, "What I am about to tell you will upset you." I immediately panicked. She told me that my uncle had been diagnosed as having HIV, the virus that causes AIDS. "He doesn't want you to know," she told me. "So don't say anything until he tells you."

I felt as though my whole world had collapsed. I was really upset and started crying but I agreed to keep quiet. What I did do was try to make it easier for him to tell me. Every time I was around him I would casually mention the topic of AIDS.

One day, about a month after my mother confided in me, my uncle and I were driving in the car and I casually mentioned that I was taking a class that discussed AIDS. I waited a few minutes to see what his reaction would be. He didn't say anything. Then I told him a few of the facts that I had learned. Again I waited. This time he said, "Did your mother tell you I have AIDS?"

I pretended that I hadn't known. But hearing it from him made it seem much more real. I was shocked but I didn't let him know. I decided to drop the subject because all of a sudden I felt uncomfortable talking about it. I had a feeling that from that day on my uncle and I would become even more close. And I was right, we have.

Last year my uncle decided to move to St. Croix for relaxation and peace. When he left it felt as though all the humor had been taken out of our family. There were no more jokes, no more gossip, nobody around to make fun of my father, no one to laugh with, and no more advice. There was also no one to help me release the stress I got from my overprotective parents.

When it finally became too much for me to bear, I got on a plane to St. Croix. When I got there, I had the time of my life. We rented a jeep and every day we went to the beach. My uncle introduced me to a friend of his who is a lesbian. What a pair they made! I remember sitting on the bed watching videos while the two of them sat there and filled me in on who was a "queen" or a "dyke." In all the years I have been in school, I have never received an education quite like the one I got on that trip.

Luckily for me, my uncle returned from St. Croix a few months ago because the family thought it would be better to have him close to home in case he got sick. He decided to go down to St. Croix every three months instead of living there year-round.

F inding out about my uncle's illness hasn't really changed our relationship. He is still the same person. The only thing that has changed is that I value the time we spend together more. Everything we do I treasure because I have learned that in life there are no guarantees. However, I still treat him the same as I always did. Maybe because I can't or don't want to fully accept what has happened.

The rest of my family has reacted a litle bit differently than I have. They've become more possessive and protective of him. These days, my poor uncle is being treated the same way my parents treat me.

My father is the worst. I understand that he is concerned about his younger brother but he tends to go overboard. One day we were in the car going to the bakery and every two minutes he would look at my uncle in the rear view mirror and ask if he was OK. I know this was getting on my uncle's nerves but he acted like it wasn't.

When the two of us go out now, the whole family tells me, "Don't keep your uncle out too long because he will get tired." I want to tell them that he is a grown man with a mind of his own, but I keep it to myself because it is none of my business. My uncle doesn't say anything.

I guess he doesn't want to hurt their feelings by telling them to get a life.

Since I found out about my uncle's diagnosis, I have become more aware of HIV and AIDS. People are dying every day, every minute. My uncle told me the best way to ensure my safety is to practice abstinence or safer sex. He told me there is not a man in the world worth dying for. I agree 100%.

Sometimes I get sad if I think about my uncle not being here. I do two things when this happens—I pray to God to protect him and then I picture him talking about somebody (usually my father) and that makes me start to laugh to myself. That makes me start to feel like he's not going anywhere.

I even told my uncle that I know he will be sitting in the first row when I graduate from high school and from college. I also informed him that he has no choice but to come to my wedding. And, knowing me and how long that will take, I can guarantee my uncle will live for a very long time.

Kia Thomas was 17 when she wrote this story.

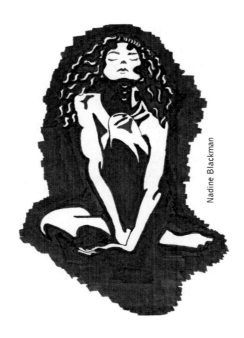

Nadine Blackman

Fear of AIDS Killed Sarah

By Christine Boose

I lost my best friend Sarah to this crazy, mysterious disease called AIDS. Yes, the same one we all think we're immune to because it only affects people who sleep around, or better yet, people who are gay.

Well, Sarah was 19. She graduated from high school and wanted to go to college to become a fashion designer. Her boyfriend Charlie was 22. They were going out for a year and four months.

Sarah was the nicest person to talk to. She always knew what to say when I was upset. She was always giving me advice, which is typical of a best friend.

Sarah didn't sleep around. She had only four boyfriends all her life, and generally, she was careful about sex. I mean, she normally used condoms, except I guess sometimes she "slipped."

Sarah called me at the end of September and told me she not only thought she was pregnant, but hoped that she was. She got a pregnancy test and was very happy to find out that, in fact, she was pregnant.

That was such a beautiful day. Charlie proposed marriage and everything. Sarah and Charlie planned to get married the day before Christmas. We were all so happy.

The next day, Sarah went to see her family doctor for a check-up. He advised her to get a complete physical, including a test for HIV (the virus that causes AIDS). When the results came back, Sarah found out she was HIV-positive. She knew that her baby was at risk of becoming HIV infected, so she decided to have an abortion. (These days, mothers who are HIV-positive can get medications to avoid passing the virus on to their babies.) Now, when I think about it, I can't believe how fast everything happened.

Until Sarah got infected, AIDS seemed so remote. However, it's actually very close to us.

Charlie also got tested and found out he was HIV-positive too.

Sarah and Charlie didn't bother blaming each other. They just went straight into a deep depression. Sarah and I saw a lot of each other then, and spoke on the phone all the time. I was the only friend that really stuck around when everybody else sort of disappeared.

Sarah was very confused. She knew too little about HIV, and she had too many questions, too many doubts, too many ugly thoughts. Since I was one of the only people she would talk to, I became very frustrated because I didn't know much about HIV myself. In other words, I didn't have all the answers and I felt very responsible.

So I decided to go for counseling at my high school, and it helped me feel better. There was an AIDS coordinator at my school who told me that it was important for Sarah to seek counseling as well, because it would help her deal with the problems she was facing as they came along.

I spoke to Sarah about how important it was that she get counseling, but she wouldn't listen. She said she didn't want to speak to anyone besides me—she didn't want to tell anyone. I also spoke with Sarah's mother and she agreed with me that counseling was important in Sarah's case, simply because we didn't know how to help her. However, all our efforts were useless.

Sarah still didn't want to speak to anyone except her mom, her boyfriend, and me. She was afraid everyone else would feel disgusted by her and reject her. She was so afraid of the stigma of AIDS and the disease itself. She felt that the time between becoming HIV infected and actually having any symptoms or even AIDS was like a rotting period. To Sarah it was all the same as death, whether it was slow or quick, painless or not. She felt she was going to die and that's all that mattered. She was obsessed.

Sarah talked a lot about killing herself. She said she lost the will to do anything since she found out she didn't have a long way to go. I didn't think she'd really do it, but I thought if I was in her position, I'd probably think about suicide too.

On the 8th of October, Sarah called me and we talked for four hours. She said she was going to do it—she wanted to kill herself that night. I didn't know what to tell her. I didn't want her to die and I told her that. But her response was, "What's the difference if I wait until I rot or just do it now!"

Poor Sarah. I wish I could have told her that so many people live for years being HIV-positive before actually getting AIDS and that there are ways of taking care of yourself, of being happy.

Sarah died that night. She took some sleeping pills, and went to sleep for good. Nobody else was in the house.

Charlie now lives with Sarah's mother in Texas. Although he's HIV-positive, he's very hopeful. He lives a normal life and while he's still very upset, he'll be all right.

I never thought much about AIDS until Sarah became HIV infected. It seemed so remote. However, AIDS is a reality. It's actually very close to us. Until Sarah, I didn't even know the difference between HIV and AIDS. Now I know that you could be infected with HIV for years, sometimes without any symptoms, before you develop full-blown AIDS. This means that if someone gets AIDS when she's in her 20s, chances are she contracted the virus in her teens.

We're all at risk—everyone who has had sexual relations without using a latex condom. We need to protect ourselves all the time, every time—not just some of the time. Sarah used protection almost every time and that wasn't good enough. Just one unsafe sexual experience can result in HIV.

I'll keep Sarah in my heart forever, but I'll also keep her in my mind to make sure I'm doing the right thing. Let Sarah be an example to every teenager. Believe me, it's very painful when you realize some sexual encounter that happened very long ago, maybe one that was not even significant enough for you to remember, can change your whole life.

Christine was 16 when she wrote this story.

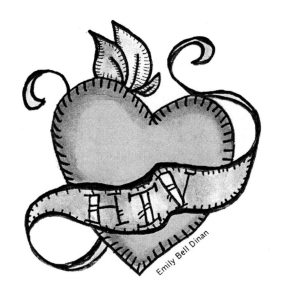

Emily Bell Dinan

The Facts About HIV and AIDS

**By Sadia Jahangir, Zaineb Nadeem, Adrian Nyxs,
Dayan Perez, and Adam Wacholder**

Even though AIDS has been around for decades now, there are still a lot of rumors and misinformation about it. We investigated some of those myths and came up with the facts. If you want more information, check out these two useful websites: **www.avert.org** and **www.gmhc.org/health/basics.html**.

Fact: You can get HIV from having unprotected sex just one time.

If you have unprotected sexual intercourse with someone who is HIV-positive, then you can get infected, even if you only do it once. And each time you have unprotected sex with an infected partner, your chances of becoming infected increase.

HIV is found in blood, semen (and pre-cum), and vaginal fluid, which is why it's risky to have sex without using a barrier—like a male or female condom—to keep partners' fluids from touching.

Fact: You can get HIV through anal sex.

Unprotected anal sex is very risky. The thin lining of the rectum is sensitive—it may allow the virus to enter the body, and it may tear, exposing blood.

Fact: You can get HIV through oral sex.

Evidence suggests a smaller risk of HIV transmission through oral sex. But it's possible to become infected with HIV through performing or receiving oral sex, especially if the giver of oral sex has cuts or sores in his or her mouth.

Fact: You can get HIV if you get a tattoo or a piercing with unsterilized instruments.

It's possible to get HIV through tattooing or body piercing, if the tools have been used on someone before you and haven't been sterilized. If you do get a tattoo or piercing, make sure the person doing it uses new or sterilized instruments.

Fact: It's possible to catch HIV from deep (French/tongue/soul) kissing—but it's not likely.

Kissing is pretty safe. While saliva might contain HIV, it's there in such small quantities that you can't possibly get infected from spit. To pick up the virus through deep kissing, blood needs to be involved, like bleeding gums or sores in the mouth. So deep kissing has a low risk of transmitting HIV.

Fact: You can get a blood transfusion without putting yourself at risk for HIV.

Although this once was a problem, the blood used for transfusions in the U.S. has been safe for many years. Donated blood gets tested for HIV before it's used. It's also safe to donate blood or have your blood drawn for medical tests.

Fact: You can't get HIV from sharing a glass or bottle.

You might catch a cold, but you won't catch HIV. HIV is not passed through saliva, or tears, or sweat.

Fact: You can't get HIV from a toilet seat.

HIV is a fragile virus that can't live long outside the body. It needs a living host. So you can't become infected from a toilet seat.

Fact: If you're HIV-positive and pregnant, medication can greatly reduce the risk of passing the virus on to your child.

A mother can pass HIV to her child before or during birth or through breast-feeding. But pregnant women who are HIV-positive can cut the risk of infecting their babies to less than 2% by taking medication and feeding their baby with formula rather than breast milk.

Fact: HIV always leads to AIDS.

HIV is a virus that breaks down the immune system, causing AIDS. It can take up to 10 years, and sometimes even longer, for HIV to do enough damage to bring on AIDS. Still, HIV will eventually lead to AIDS.

Fact: If you've been infected with HIV, it may not show up on a test right away.

The most readily available test for HIV looks for the existence of antibodies (cells that form in reaction to the virus). It usually takes about three months after the virus enters the system for the body to make enough antibodies to show up on the test. (In rare cases, it can take up to six months for the antibodies to show up.) So it's best to wait at least three months after your possible exposure to get tested—and be careful not to do anything in the meantime that might infect someone else.

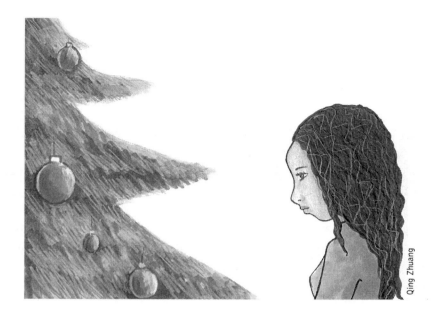

Suffering in Silence

By Diane Brandon

I remember Thanksgiving 2002. That was the last Thanksgiving I ever spent with my older brother David. At the time I didn't know it was going to be his last Thanksgiving, since he was only 33 years old. I treated it like any other holiday with my family, eating and spending time together.

Then Christmas Eve came. My mother walked into my bedroom and told me that we had to go to the hospital because David was sick. She looked really worried but she didn't say why. I expected to hear that whatever he had wasn't too serious.

My mother and I went to see him that night. I thought that he just had a bad cold, but he looked really thin. It wasn't until later that night, when my mother and I came home, that she told me what she'd learned that day—that my brother had AIDS.

I didn't know how I felt. I think I was in shock. I was 12 years old and I didn't know as many things about AIDS as I know now. But I knew that it can be transmitted through sex and that people can die from it (I learned later that AIDS can also be transmitted when people using drugs share needles).

I asked my mother what was going to happen to my brother. I wanted to know how he'd gotten AIDS, how long he'd had it, and was he going to die? I wanted to know if the hospital could do anything to stop him from dying. I kept hoping that the doctors had made a mistake or maybe they got his forms mixed up with another person.

But my mother couldn't answer most of my questions because they were her questions too. So I stopped asking and stayed quiet. That Christmas felt really slow and unreal and I just couldn't get the thought out of my head that my brother was about to die.

My mother tried to be cheerful, like she usually is on holidays. The living room was decorated with a Christmas tree, flashing colored lights, and candy canes. It looked like Christmas but it didn't feel like Christmas.

Part of me was expecting David to pull through, just like in the movies.

She tried to not break down even though she must have been taking his sickness the hardest. I didn't know how to console her so I didn't do anything. Most of the time I stayed in my room to avoid contact with her, but when I was near her I tried to act normal. I talked to my friends on the phone, played with my cat, and watched TV.

My mom, one of my other brothers and I took a cab to the hospital on Christmas Day, which didn't make us feel any better. The whole hospital vibe felt bad. It made me think of death, despite the Christmas decorations everywhere. The hospital was painted an odd mint green, and it smelled like sick people. The place gave me the chills.

I wanted to be at home at our apartment in Manhattan, watching Christmas shows, with the Christmas lights reflecting off the wall. Being in a hospital was not my idea of Christmas.

I did want to see David but I didn't want him to be in the hospital. He was too skinny and he looked like he was in pain even though he was asleep most of the time. None of us talked. We just sat in his room and looked at him sleeping.

I never bothered to talk to my friends, my mother, or my other two brothers about David. I thought that if I didn't talk about it, then it wouldn't be true. I still saw my friends at school and talked with them on the phone about school or boys.

I felt like I needed to act normal. It was my attempt to fool myself into thinking everything was OK. Other than going to school, I mostly stayed in my room—but that was normal for me too. I tried my hardest not to do anything differently.

But I did write about my feelings in my journal. I'd started a journal a little bit before I found out about my brother's disease. It was a black book that I wrote in whenever I was mad or disappointed, a book for all my anger and sadness.

I separated my good, happy entries and my gloomy, disappointed entries. I wrote almost every day for more than a month. Although I probably needed someone to talk to, I felt like paper was the only thing that understood me at that time.

I wrote all about David, about how I didn't understand why he didn't protect himself, about whether he'd still be able to protect me without actually being here and whether he was still happy.

I never did fully realize that my brother wasn't going to make it, and I'm not sure my mother did either. When a character in a movie is supposed to die, he or she always seems to get better. Part of me was expecting David to pull through, just like in the movies.

Of my three brothers (all older than me), he was the one I saw the most. He only lived a block away, and he was always at my house. He'd eat with us or have a snack and watch TV. I'd gotten so used to seeing him at my apartment or outside when I came home from school. When he wasn't around anymore, I couldn't believe it.

The day he died was hard, really hard. My mother and I were home when someone from the hospital called and told her that her son hadn't made it.

I was sitting in my room when I heard my mother's loud cries. I walked into her room to see what had happened and she told me. I just stood there and stared at her. None of that night or the next day felt real. I kept hoping I'd wake up from this nightmare.

The wake and the funeral were very classy, but that didn't matter. My brother was still in a casket and that was when the reality hit me hard. Everything my mother had told me was true. My brother really did have AIDS and he really had died from it.

When I saw everyone crying, I just froze. I thought I had no more emotion left to feel. During the few weeks that I'd known about his disease, I'd tried to block all my emotions and that took a lot out of me. When I wanted to let it all go and cry at his funeral, the feelings wouldn't come out.

I thought that if I didn't talk about it, then it wouldn't be true.

But when I was walking up the aisle to the exit at the funeral, I felt everyone looking at me with those sad "I'm sorry" eyes. That's when I broke down in front of everyone. My emotions took over and I started to cry. Then I got mad because people were looking at me and trying to console me. I didn't want to be consoled. I wanted to just cry.

When we went to the gravesite, it was so hard to see my brother being lowered into the ground. That was going to be the last time I ever saw his body. I felt numb, just standing there and watching.

Three years after his death, I still don't know or understand all the choices he made. Maybe he chose to have unprotected sex, but I'll probably never find out. He might not even have known how he got AIDS. I wish that I knew more.

My mother told me he eventually refused to take his medication after he found out he was sick. I wish he had taken the medication so maybe he could still be here.

I miss my brother always hanging out at the house and being protective of me. I always felt safe when I was with him. I know that wishing won't make him come back, but I still do it. I still hope that in some impossible way, he'll come back.

Diane was 16 when she wrote this story.

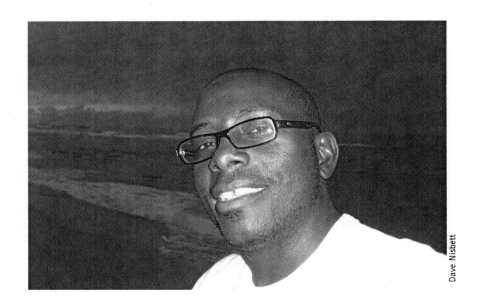

Dave Nisbett

Twenty Years Living Positive

By Orubba Almansouri, Natasha Dawkins, Marsha Dupiton, Keenen Freeman, Courtney Smith, and Divine Strickland

Dave Nisbett contracted HIV 20 years ago, when he was 15. Back then, the diagnosis still amounted to a death sentence for many. But Nisbett has never let his diagnosis stop him from living his life. He's a single father to three daughters, and divides his time between being a stay-at-home dad, blogging about his life, and going to college, where he's double majoring in political science and philosophy. We spoke to him about what it's been like to live with HIV for so long.

Q: How did you find out that you had HIV?

A: When I was 18, in January 1991, I was trying to get into the

Marines, and an HIV test was required for entry. My recruiter actually told my grandmother I was positive before he told me. I confronted the recruiter and he said, "You need to get your blood checked. I don't know what else to tell you."

Q: Do you know how you got infected?

A: I was 15, living in North Carolina with my parents and sister. I had just come out to them as bisexual. My father didn't take it well, and it was a traumatic experience. There was all this tension in the house and I just wanted to get out.

One Saturday, I took a walk in the park and had an unprotected same-sex encounter with a stranger. I knew about HIV and how to protect myself, but I didn't think about what I was putting myself at risk for.

Right after the encounter I got anal warts, an STD. At the emergency room, the doctor who treated me didn't mention anything about HIV. Eventually it went away and I tried to block it out of my mind.

But three years later when the HIV test results came back from the Marines, I knew that was the encounter that had infected me.

Q: What did you do when you found out you were positive?

A: When I got off the phone with the recruiter, I remember just staring at the phone, like, "What am I gonna do now?" All sorts of thoughts were running through my head about living and dying. At that time there was an ad campaign with the national AIDS hotline number, and since the phone was right there I said, "You know what? Let me just call." I called and was immediately referred to an adolescent clinic in the Bronx.

My girlfriend at the time was the first person I told after that. She and I were intimate and even though we had protected sex, it was important that I tell her. She was wonderful. She said, "Do you want me to go with you to the clinic?" We went and they explained what the risk factors were. We eventually broke up, but not because of my status.

Then I had a conversation with my grandmother. The family was worried about whether it was safe to have me in the apartment because my sister was pregnant (she and I both lived with my grandmother). The adolescent clinic brought us all in for family counseling and explained what the risks were and weren't. They did a great job of educating us.

My parents were in North Carolina and I told them over the phone. My dad didn't show much emotion, but my mom was crying and saying how sorry she was. The following summer she came up to New York and I remember her being really cautious around me. One day I saw her secretly disinfecting the toilet after I'd used the bathroom.

Q: Were you able to get the right treatment for your disease?

A: Had I not made that phone call right away and gotten the referral to the adolescent clinic at Montefiore Medical Center in the Bronx, I think my life would have turned out differently. In 1991 it was only the second adolescent HIV clinic in the country. The support services that they have there, I couldn't ask for more.

It wasn't until 2003 that my immune system started to decline enough for me to be diagnosed with AIDS and have to go on medication, leave my job, and go on disability. So for 12 years I was doing my thing—I had a career as a case manager for other HIV-affected families, got married and had kids.

I've been on the same treatment regimen since 2004. I get side effects like upset stomach; I have to eat before I take the medicine. But it's the fatigue that gets me most of the time. I take four to five pills once a day. It's intense because if I take it at 11:00 a.m., I have to maintain that. If 11 a.m. the next day comes and I don't take my medicine, the HIV virus will say, "There's no medicine here, let's cause some havoc." That's how your viral load rises and your T cell count declines.

Q: How did you have three children and keep them HIV-free?

A: When I met my wife in 1997 (we've since separated), I told her immediately that I was bisexual and HIV-positive. We just fell in love; it was such a soul-mate thing. After we'd been together for about four or five months we started to talk about having kids.

My doctor said, "That's really risky." But I've always had a low viral load and a high T cell count, which suggests that at any given time there isn't a lot of HIV in my blood and semen. It was an intense decision to make, but we stopped having protected sex to conceive, and as soon as we found out she was pregnant we went back to protected sex.

My kids see the medicine I take every day. They know there are good days and bad days

It's a crazy thing to say, but she was willing to risk becoming infected for us to have a family together. She had to take three HIV tests during both pregnancies (she already had our oldest daughter from a previous relationship) and then another right before delivery to make sure she wasn't infected. All those tests came back negative. If she had become infected, they would have given her medication to prevent the baby from being infected during childbirth.

Q: Did you tell your daughters about your disease?

A: My oldest is 14 and I have a 9-year-old and an 8-year-old. Our relationship is incredible; we talk about everything. I told them the whole story in age-appropriate terms. I told them I'm bisexual almost four years ago. Gradually I started introducing HIV into our conversations and got some books about HIV. Then I told them somebody in our family had HIV, and that I wasn't going to tell them who it was yet. Almost a year later, in December, 2007, I told them it was me.

They were surprised. My 14-year-old (she was 13 at the time) wanted to know, "Does that mean Mommy is positive? Does that mean we are?" I felt really fortunate to be able to say to them that, no, they and Mommy weren't infected.

It's an ongoing conversation. I didn't want to just drop it at the dinner table and say, "OK, don't ask Daddy about it again." They see the medicine I take every day. They know there are good days and bad days.

Q: How do you balance managing your disease and being a single father to three girls?

A: They're with me four days a week and with their mom three days a week. They have lots of friends who don't have fathers in their lives or have the routine that we have. I pick them up from school. We do homework. I cook, I clean. We have dinner together at 5:30.

The only time it's irregular is when I don't feel well, physically or emotionally—I also suffer from depression, which I think has been more debilitating to me over the years than the physical symptoms of HIV. When that happens, I take care of responsibilities but then I rest, and they see Daddy's a little quiet, a little subdued. Before they knew I had HIV and depression it was hard for them to understand why Daddy is up sometimes and down sometimes. Now that they know, they're able to say, "Daddy's not feeling well today; let's just chill out." I always tell them when they see me down, "Tomorrow's another day."

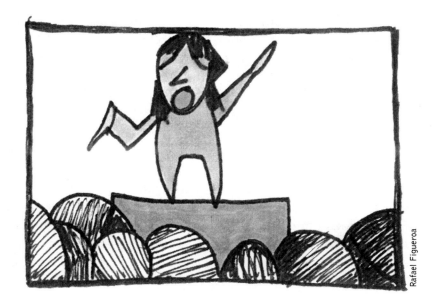

Rafael Figueroa

Acting Is My Activism

By Marsha Dupiton

As my friends and I filed down the aisle of our high school auditorium, there they stood: a group of teens all in identical black shirts and jeans, in two parallel lines with their heads down.

"What, are they going to step?" I whispered to my friend.

She chuckled and directed her attention to the stage. I rolled my eyes and waited. When everyone was quiet, one of the performers yelled out, "Being frisky can be risky!" Everyone laughed, and I was hooked.

THEO (Teens Helping Each Other) is a Brooklyn, NY-based peer education project. Paid teen participants use improvisational theater to educate other teens at schools, churches, and community programs about HIV and other STDs. On weekday afternoons in the THEO office in Crown Heights, Brooklyn, teen participants get down to work, after-school style.

When I saw the group perform at my school that day in 10th grade, the funny slogans about unprotected sex were followed by a 15-minute skit about a sexually active teen couple, where the girl got an STD from the boy. The girl and boy portrayed real emotion, as if this was something they were really going through. I could relate to their conversation, unlike if they had just spit out tons of sex education material.

Afterward, when the program coordinator came onstage and offered students applications to join the program, I took one right away. I was already in the theater club in my school and I really liked acting. I was also interested in educating my peers about a serious topic like HIV and other STDs. The performers I saw weren't afraid to talk about things many people keep quiet about, and I thought they were brave. I was shy and I wanted to learn how to gain the respect and trust of an audience the way the performers had.

As a trainee at THEO, I spent a summer learning about HIV and other STDs and about human anatomy and physiology. We were even responsible for a "baby" (a doll) over the summer, an activity that showed us the difficulty of being a teen parent.

One thing I found interesting was learning some of the common myths about HIV. For instance, when HIV first appeared, many people thought only gay men were able to contract the disease. It wasn't until a highly publicized case of a young boy getting HIV from a tainted blood transfusion in 1984 that people began to realize that anyone can get the virus. Now we know that HIV does not have a particular face or race. (Nearly half the people newly infected in 2006 were heterosexual, according to the Centers for Disease Control.)

The first time I performed after my training was exhilarating. It was at a church in front of more than 300 people whose eyes were all on me and my fellow peer educators. We performed "Sistas in the Hood," a skit where several girls are pressuring their friend to have sex. I had to "be" my character:

loud, ghetto, and aggressive, someone who sleeps with a lot of people and pressures her friend to do the same.

At first this was difficult because the character was so different from me. I also had to be quick, clever, and funny with my responses because the whole thing was improvised. When we perform, we are given a scenario that sets up the scene for us, but the dialogue is completely up to us. There is no writing down scripts or memorizing lines. We have to make up our lines on the spot, letting the words flow and the feeling shine right out of us.

To help us learn how to get into character and improvise, our supervisor had us do different exercises, like a character walk. We would go around the room in a big circle, trying to walk like our character and get in the character's mindset. Eventually

The performers I saw weren't afraid to talk about things many people keep quiet about.

I got better at improvising and I didn't need to do the character walk before every performance or rehearsal.

The point of our performances is to give the audience a visual of the daily pressures that teens experience, what can happen when you have unprotected sex, and how HIV and other STDs can affect someone's life. Our skits help the audience relate to the topic at hand. After we do the skit, we sometimes discuss the topic with the audience or give basic information about HIV, like how it can be contracted, how you can protect yourself and the treatment for it.

Then, we ask teens in the audience what they think. They usually say they can relate to the skit and that they feel that we've given them more of an understanding of the HIV epidemic. That feels good.

Being in THEO for two and a half years has contributed to my life in many ways. I know that I have a second support system and family. I've also become more mature, partly because I'm responsible for showing newcomers the ropes. And I love acting and talking to my peers about an epidemic that threatens our city and our world each and every day.

When I finish my time at THEO at the end of this year, I feel like I will have made an impact on many of my peers. And to me that is the greatest reward.

Marsha was 17 when she wrote this story. After graduating from high school she enrolled in Ithaca College.

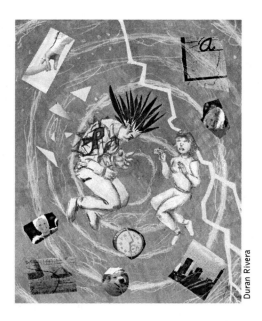

Duran Rivera

My Dad Has HIV

By Anonymous

Whenever I'm sick, I watch an old movie in my DVD collection. Last month, when I was home with the flu, I pulled out Forrest Gump, a movie that never made me cry—until now.

I got up to the part when Forrest's friend Jenny is in bed, dying from AIDS. She couldn't get up and finally she died. That got me bawling and I couldn't help thinking, "What if Daddy got like this? When will Daddy get like this?"

My dad was diagnosed with HIV two years ago. He takes several pills a day to keep the disease from becoming a threat. I pray the medicines never stop working, but what if they do? What if the virus develops resistance to them? He could end up like Jenny.

The day my father told me he had HIV, he was sitting down on the love seat in the living room, and I was sitting at the computer, as usual. My mother had stepped out of the room. He called me over and told me to sit by him. I sat down on the floor beside the coffee table.

He said very bluntly, "Sweetie, I have HIV." I stammered, but couldn't reply. Finally I caught my speech and asked him if he was all right. He nodded, but we both started to cry.

I was more than shocked. I mean, I never thought about this happening to someone in my family. Contracting HIV only happens to drug addicts and sex fiends, right? No. It can happen to every kind of person. Even my Daddy.

My dad, who works in a hospital as a building service supervisor, told me that years earlier, he'd been stuck with a needle while tossing something in the laboratory trash. Someone had thrown the needle in the wrong garbage can. My dad explained that the tests the doctors gave him at the time didn't show that he had HIV.

Contracting HIV only happens to drug addicts and sex fiends, right?

He realized he needed to see the doctor again when he developed a strange rash on his chest, 11 years later. The doctor told him he had thrush. Thrush is an opportunistic disease, which means that it can only attack babies and those with weak immune systems. This set an alarm off in the doctor's head and my father was tested for HIV. When my dad tested positive, the doctor put him on a regimen of drugs.

After my dad told me, I went in my room, bawling, and shut my door. I put my music up so he wouldn't hear me crying. I couldn't believe my father was sick with a deadly disease. It was terrible to come to terms with. I didn't want to acknowledge it. I wanted to pretend it didn't exist, but I had to realize it was there. It was killing my daddy.

I couldn't look him in the eye that day for fear of breaking down in tears. I didn't want to hurt him or make him feel awkward. I didn't want to make him feel bad for telling me, like it was the wrong thing to do.

I wanted to prove to Daddy (and maybe myself) that I was strong enough to handle this, and that I could be there for him without crying like a baby. But I was pretty distraught.

After my father broke the news to my sister, he told us both that we weren't allowed to tell anyone about the disease—not friends, family, or teachers. My father didn't want anyone to look at him differently, and he didn't want us to be looked upon differently.

We swore we wouldn't tell anyone about him being sick. But I was extremely worried that his health and life was in danger. And I needed to let my closest friends know how I felt.

So I turned Daddy into "Cousin Louis." The next day at school, I told my friend Diana that "Louis," the cousin I was so very close to, had told me he was HIV-positive the night before. She sighed and hugged me. But I didn't want pity, I wanted a listening ear.

Diana's boyfriend, my other closest friend at the time, lent me that ear, asking me how he contracted the disease. I told him how "Louis" had caught it. He nodded and took me from Diana, letting me sob into his shoulder, murmuring more of the situation.

I never told my dad that I told them. I'm still afraid he's worried about what people might think of him.

Nowadays, most of my friends never hear me voice my fears. I only tell Diana and her boyfriend when I'm really concerned about my father. (I slipped and told them last summer that "Louis" was my dad.) But I'm always afraid I'll burden them with my worries—and I don't want them worrying about me. I don't think my worries should be placed on anyone else's shoulders. Instead, I write them down in a book.

Some things haven't changed much since my dad was diagnosed with HIV. We have a typical father-(teenage) daughter relationship. We fight from time to time, but I always come back and tell him I love him. Then I ask for money.

I rarely think about his condition day-to-day, but when I do, I just feel like falling. The other day he cut himself and I wanted to help so badly, but he refused to let me clean or bandage him, in case I had an open wound or cut on my hand somewhere I didn't know about.

Before my father had HIV, he rarely got sick. He was energetic, lively, and strong. He was everyone's rock. Now he gets sick at a drop of a hat. Yet he still goes to work. Only immediate management knows he has HIV because he doesn't want to be discriminated against.

Still, when there's a cold in the house, he almost always automatically gets it. I always feel guilty when he gets sick because it makes me think, "Did I give that to him?" So every time I have a cold, I try to steer clear of Daddy.

> *I rarely think about my dad's condition day-to-day, but when I do, I just feel like falling.*

I think being sick scares Daddy. It would scare me. I think he's become more insecure about himself. He worries more about life and his job. He often talks about our financial situation if, God forbid, he dies. The double shifts at work are hard for him now, but he puts himself through them anyway because he's devoted to taking care of us.

I wish I could take care of him the way he takes care of us. I hope he never has to depend on me like that, though. I don't want him to ever have to be dependent on anyone. I want him to always be healthy and strong enough to be independent.

But even though he gets sick more easily now than before, he's still in pretty good shape. His white blood count is up and the viral load is down, which means his body is doing a good job of fighting the virus.

He's on an anti-viral regimen, which is a group of medicines that battle the disease because the immune system is unable to. He's responded to it well, though his doctors change his pills frequently so the virus doesn't develop resistance to the medicines.

I'm scared that one day his drugs will stop working and he'll die. It chills my bones to think about all the people who've become resistant to their drug regimen and just withered away. I pray it never happens to my father.

I sometimes think about how much my dad means to me. I think every girl needs her daddy. He comforts me when I'm sad, lectures me when I've done something wrong, and helps me figure out problems.

I have no idea what I'd do if Daddy ever passed away. I don't think I could handle not having my dad. It's just too painful for my heart to grasp.

The author was in high school when she wrote this story.

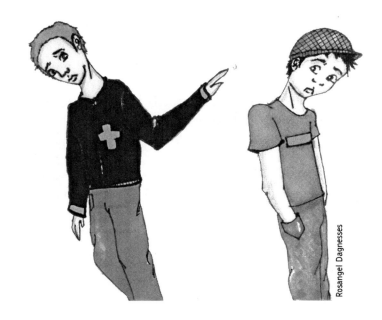

Rosangel Dagnesses

Too Big a Risk

By Anonymous

After my first boyfriend and I broke up, it tore me up inside. When I learned that he had a new boyfriend just four months later, I knew I had to get over him and make a new beginning with someone else, too. I guess you could say I was looking for a "rebound" boyfriend. What I ended up with was a situation I never thought I would have to go through.

While browsing through my friend's MySpace page one day, I found the page of a cute boy I had seen around but never spoken to. It was crazy; we would always stare into each other's eyes when we saw each other with our mutual friends, but we never said a thing.

I sent him a friend request and waited, nervous that he would decline it. To my surprise, he accepted. We began to write

MySpace messages to each other and later started instant messaging. We would chat online all day long.

Ray was 20, two years older than me, and he was the nicest guy I had met since my ex. We talked about our dreams, goals, life experiences, and past relationships. Soon, we were talking on the phone every night, sometimes until the sun came up. I began to have strong feelings for him.

One night, I decided to pick Ray up from work. We had seen each other before, but this was the first time it was just the two of us. We talked and held hands like a couple. When he asked me if I wanted to come to his house, I said yes without hesitation.

At his house, where he lived with some roommates, we took off our clothes and lay in his bed. He massaged my back and we talked a little, but the conversation got interrupted when Ray gave me a kiss on the lips. I was scared and unsure if I was ready to move on to the next guy just yet. But I dismissed my doubts when I looked into Ray's eyes. We kissed for a while and then called it a night, falling asleep in each other's arms.

The next morning, Ray made me breakfast in bed—scrambled eggs with cheese, bacon, grits, pancakes, and apple juice. He ironed my clothes for me and walked me to the train. I felt so special. It felt like we were actually in a relationship.

Then, as the train was approaching the station, Ray suddenly said, "I think that you should live your life and do you." He basically meant that I should find someone else to be with. I was confused and hurt. Why did he suddenly feel this way about me? What had I done?

I didn't hear from Ray for an entire week. Seven days felt like seven months. Finally, when I came home from the store one day, my mother told me that Ray had called. I dialed his number, happy but at the same time scared.

When he answered the phone, he sounded depressed, and he said he had to tell me something very important.

"You are so special to me and I don't ever want to see you

hurt again, but you and I are two different types of people," he said.

I thought, "This can't be happening to me again. Why doesn't anyone want to be in a relationship with me?" After about a minute of total silence, I asked, "What do you mean, we're two different types of people?"

He just said that he needed some time to think and he would call me later.

A few days later, I called Ray and asked him again what he had meant.

"Disease," was the only word that came out of his mouth.

"What the heck is this boy talking about?" I thought nervously.

Ray said he was on his lunch break out in public and he didn't want to say it out loud. He told me to name some diseases and when I named the right one he would say yes. I remembered Ray telling me about all the wild sexual things he'd done with guys in the past, and I began to name all of the STDs I could think of, from genital herpes to syphilis.

Finally, I said, "AIDS," praying that he would reject my guess. I took a deep breath and waited for his answer.

"Not that, but the stage that comes before it," Ray said. That's how I found out that Ray was HIV-positive.

I was shocked and hurt, but I also felt sympathetic toward Ray. I didn't know what to say to him. All I could do was cry and think of how grateful I was to not be in his position. "Don't worry, I'm going to be here for you," was all I managed to say.

Ray talked about his day-to-day struggles, his medication, and how he felt about the whole situation. Later, he said he thought there would be no problem with us being in a relationship, but he would feel very nervous when it came to us being sexual with each other. That's why he had stopped calling me for a week.

I wasn't sure what to do. I had strong feelings for Ray and the last thing I wanted was to leave him right when he needed me most. But I told him I would be scared about the sexual part, too. He said he would not want to be a burden on me, and that he would feel awful if he passed his HIV to me. We agreed to continue getting to know each other, with the possibility of a relationship later.

But as the weeks passed, Ray started to distance himself from me. Before, he would call me many times a day. Now he would only call once a day, around midnight. I basically felt like he had given up on us because he was afraid that he would give me HIV.

I began to name all of the STDs I could think of, from genital herpes to syphilis. Finally, I said, "AIDS."

I never gave up on him, though. I continued to call, no matter how many times I got his voicemail. Even though I wasn't sure I could handle being with someone who was HIV-positive, I wanted to prove to Ray that I could do it. I began to do research on the Internet to see how it might be possible to date him.

I educated myself more about HIV and learned that many things I had thought were true were actually just myths. I found out that you can't catch HIV from kissing someone or from drinking from the same glass as someone with HIV.

But I also learned that I wouldn't be able to handle dating someone who is HIV-positive. Even if you use a condom, there's still a possibility that you could contract the disease, and that felt like too big a risk. I still have feelings for Ray, but I've decided to just be his friend. I never told Ray my decision and he hasn't asked. We just talk to each other as friends now.

I feel like people with HIV should give potential partners who are HIV-negative the chance to choose whether they want to be in a relationship with them or not, the way Ray did with me.

It might be hard to deal with the rejection if the person decides not to be with you because you have HIV, but it's still the right thing to do. I'm grateful that Ray was honest with me. And even though I decided not to date him, Ray has a place in my heart and I will always be there for him when he needs me.

The author was 18 when he wrote this story.

•

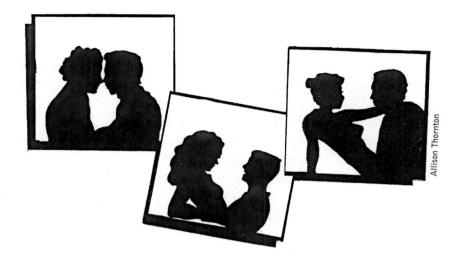

Allison Thornton

There's More to Sex Than Sex

By Anonymous

Humping, fingering, jerking off, rubbing, petting, licking, suck-ing, stroking, first base, second base, third base, foreplay, kissing, hugging, necking, making out....Call it what you want, there is a whole other world outside of sexual intercourse.

"People do a lot of crazy stuff before they do it," said David, 17.

But why not do the crazy stuff instead of doing "it"? Especially if you don't have a condom, you're afraid of AIDS, pregnancy, or nasty things like genital warts—or if you're just not ready.

People often overlook things like kissing, hugging, even holding hands. "Anything can be erotic and enormously satisfy-ing," said Andy Humm of the Hetrick-Martin Institute. "Sex is more than intercourse...It's more than doing the deed: the thing is in, the thing is out."

Humm recommends that teens use their imaginations. There are many ways of expressing yourself sexually other than intercourse.

"Humping" is about the closest you can get without putting yourself or your partner at significant risk of catching a sexually transmitted disease (STD) or getting pregnant. That's when two people rub their pelvic areas together simulating intercourse but the penis does not penetrate the vagina. It can be done with or without your clothes on (although without clothes you have to be careful no semen or vaginal fluids are exchanged).

There are many ways of expressing yourself sexually other than intercourse.

People also use their hands to stroke, finger, and "jerk" each other. This is also known as mutual masturbation.

There are still some small risks that come with these alternatives. Even without having intercourse you or your partner can contract chlamydia, herpes, or pubic lice (crabs), for example, just through genital contact.

What about HIV, the virus which causes AIDS? "Theoretically, if you rub too hard, there is a risk," said Teri Lewis, director of the AIDS and Adolescents Network of New York, "but people always have these 'What ifs?'"

Any cuts, open sores, or conditions such as poison ivy might pose a small risk if you choose to engage in mutual masturbation because they are potential passageways for infection.

There have been studies claiming that about 25% of all teenagers have engaged in anal sex, often to avoid pregnancy or preserve their virginity. But anal sex is not a safe alternative since there is a higher risk of catching HIV even with a condom. During anal sex, there is a greater chance that the condom will break and that tissue will tear even if you don't see any blood.

The risks of STDs and unwanted pregnancy can be avoided if you choose an alternative to intercourse. Michael has done some "other stuff" because he did not have a condom But he adds: "If we had a condom, we would have done it."

If you're not ready for intercourse, but you think that you might be ready for some of the alternatives, there are some other things you should think about as well. Not everybody is ready for what experts call "outercourse" either.

"You have to ask yourself, 'Can I handle this?'" says Lewis. "'Do I trust this person?', 'Can I speak to this person?'"

Some people can't trust themselves; once they get started, they can't stop themselves after a certain point. For some people only intercourse counts as real sex. Still others won't engage in any type of sexual activity until they are married. "There's no rush," said Ana, 17.

You have to decide for yourself what you think is right for you. Whether you choose to have intercourse, outercourse, or to remain abstinent, the most important thing is to talk about the decision with your partner.

There might be a point where you would like to stop. Say you don't want to do anything beyond French kissing, for example. According to Lewis, the two of you have to work that out together—ahead of time: "You have to decide that 'We won't get further.'"

But what if your partner disagrees with you? "Ask yourself the hard question, 'Is this the relationship that I want?'" Lewis cautions. "If you can't reach compromises about this then you probably can't reach others."

The author wrote this story when she was in high school.
She went on to college and studied art history.

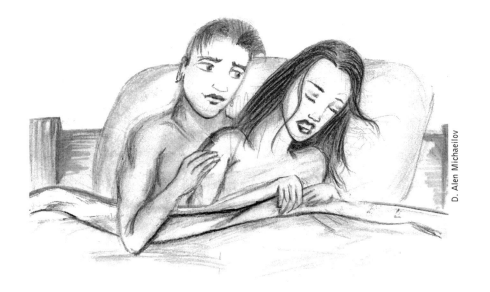

No Excuse Is Good Enough

By Mimi Callaghan

How come some teens still don't use protection? We all know the dangers of having unprotected sex. We all know that we can end up getting diseases like herpes, gonorrhea, syphilis, and HIV if we don't use a condom. And then there's what we always seem to forget: girls can get pregnant.

I asked different people, male and female, ages 14-22, why they did and didn't use condoms. Below are the answers they gave me, and some information about why their excuses could get them in a lot of trouble.

1. "I haven't gotten sick."

Many STDs have no symptoms the first few months, so you can't be sure you haven't gotten sick.

Just because you're not deathly ill doesn't mean you don't

have an STD. Chlamydia and gonorrhea often don't have symptoms. But for many women, they turn into PID (pelvic inflammatory disease).

PID can make girls infertile, which means they can never have children. In the short term, PID gives girls chronic pelvic pain, and many girls with PID have to be hospitalized.

Also, AIDS doesn't usually have symptoms until years after infection. Someone could have HIV and look perfectly fine.

Plus, people with syphilis, gonorrhea, chlamydia, or herpes are two to five times more likely than others to get infected with HIV. That is pretty frightening.

So even if you and your partner feel fine, you need to be careful.

2. "I'd use a condom if the guy wanted to."

You're in control of your own life and your own body. And if not, then you're in a very unhealthy relationship.

Why make the guy decide if you should protect yourself, especially since he isn't the one who can get pregnant? And if you do get pregnant, the guy won't always stick around.

Now don't get me wrong. I know there are guys who stay and support their kids. I know a few guys who take care of their kids and that's great. However, most of the time, that isn't the case.

I asked Matt Apple, a college student, what he would do if his girlfriend got pregnant. His response was, "Abort! Abort! Abandon ship!" Now, what if he was your boyfriend?

Most girls feel like: "I am too young to have a child and I don't know if I could handle an abortion."

If you feel that way, you need to plan ahead and use birth control.

3. "I know we're both clean."

STDs are easily contracted. You never know who might have these diseases. And if your girlfriend or boyfriend cheats on you just once, she or he might contract an STD. Especially since 20-40% of sexually active teens have chlamydia.

And you can't always take just one test and say you're fine. HIV doesn't show up in your bloodstream for three to six months after infection.

Not only that, but you can get really gross diseases like herpes, which has had a 30% increase of cases since the 1970s. One in five Americans older than 12 is infected with genital herpes.

Would you risk your life for one good orgasm?

And I know for a fact that people lie about how many people they have been with. I have a friend who told her beau that she had slept with five people, when the real number was in the teens.

Another friend of mine slept with a girl and told her that she was his first. But I knew the girl he lost his virginity to.

The fact is, you should not trust anyone with your health and your life. They might be lying so you don't think differently of them because they have been with multiple partners.

You can't tell by looking at somebody what they have. They can look completely healthy, but they can still get you sick.

4. "If I was with someone who was really hot and didn't want to use one, I'd say OK."

That's pretty frightening, since we usually sleep with people we are attracted to.

5. "It doesn't feel as good."

As my friend Stephanie said: "Would you risk your life for one good orgasm? No."

6. "I know when to pull out."

A friend of mine used to tell me how she hates the feel of condoms and how much better it is that her boyfriend doesn't wear one.

Her protection against pregnancy was the "pull-out method," which is when your partner pulls out before he ejaculates.

She took back those words when she was three months late with her period and her boyfriend of a year had been cheating on her. So much for her pull-out method.

Things squirt in there, you know, even though you don't feel it. There is that pre-cum stuff.

And Planned Parenthood warns teens especially against using this method, because teenage boys aren't very good at knowing when to pull out. They don't have as much experience with how their bodies work, and they're also likely to prematurely ejaculate.

7. "Don't you trust me?" or "What, do you think I am dirty?"

If your partner says, "Don't you trust me?" you should say, "What are you talking about? Pregnancy and disease has nothing to do with trust."

Come on, there is a 90% chance that girls who don't use contraceptives for one year will wind up pregnant. The numbers are frightening.

The final word is: If someone doesn't want to use a condom, then that person doesn't respect you or your body.

If you're having unprotected sex, you're taking more of a chance than you may think.

Now, I admit that I have been stupid and have not used protection every time. I know my reasons were not good enough. There is no excuse.

I didn't care about what happened, and I knew the person only slept with one other person. Later on, I realized I couldn't be too sure about that. Thankfully, we both were clean, and I didn't get pregnant. I was lucky. I'm not proud about what happened. The fact of the matter is, I protect myself now.

If teens are told something too much, they turn it off. Like when your mom tells you to clean your room, you just don't because you're tired of hearing it. In some ways, I think teens don't use protection because they're rebelling.

Rebellion is not a good reason to leave your condoms home, just as all the other excuses my friends told me weren't good reasons either.

What I'm trying to say is, why risk it? Yes, we're all human and we all mess up, but it's easy enough to protect ourselves. If you're having unprotected sex, you're taking more of a chance than you may think.

Mimi was 17 when she wrote this story. She graduated high school and studied forensic psychology in college.

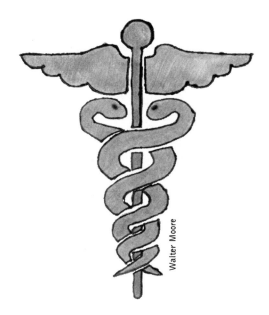

Walter Moore

HIV: Still Searching for a Cure

By Courtney Smith

Have you ever wondered whether someone will find a cure for HIV, the virus that causes AIDS?

In 2008, the Wall Street Journal reported on a new development in the search for a cure. An HIV-positive American man who lived in Germany had received a bone marrow transplant to treat leukemia, and two years after the surgery, his body showed no trace of HIV.

But doctors are wary of calling this case a "cure," because there were at least 32 attempts to rid people of HIV this way between 1982 and 1996, and only two seemed to succeed. Many developments have brought new hope in the field of AIDS research, but it's still a deadly disease without a vaccine or known cure.

Since the general public became aware of HIV and AIDS in

the 1980s, treatments for the virus have helped make the disease more manageable. AZT, the first drug approved for treating HIV, came out in 1987. AZT prevents HIV from changing its RNA, or genetic material, into DNA. (Once it changes its RNA into DNA, the virus can "instruct" the human cell it has infected to make more of the virus.)

At first, AZT didn't help much, because it has to be taken before HIV "takes over" an infected cell's genetic material. It did reduce the risk of mothers passing the virus to babies during childbirth and breast feeding, though, and infant HIV infections began to decrease.

Combination antiretroviral treatment, which is a treatment that uses more than one type of drug, was developed in 1996 and is highly effective against HIV. It isn't a cure, but it can prevent people from becoming ill for many years. The treatment includes multiple pills that have to be taken every day. The drugs keep the presence of HIV in the body at a low level, which stops the immune system from weakening and lets it recover from the damage the HIV virus has done already.

Finding out you have HIV today doesn't mean you will die tomorrow—in fact, many people now live long, healthy lives with it. But that's not a guarantee. To keep your immune system strong you'll have to take many pills, which have to be taken in very specific ways and often have side effects. You'll face telling potential sex partners about your HIV status, and it may influence your decisions about having a family.

Some scientists are working on developing a vaccine against HIV. However, there are no guarantees. In 2003, one experimental vaccine underwent a trial but was found ineffective. In 2007, another HIV vaccine was attempted, but it showed no benefits.

Despite all the promising new research, no one can be sure that we will have a solid vaccine or cure in the future. The best prevention for HIV is still abstinence or using condoms. It's important to have good communication and honesty with a potential sex partner about your sexual history and whether you've both been tested. But in the end, having sex without a condom is a big risk, no matter what is said or how long you've been with a person.

Courtney was 18 when she wrote this story.

Getting Tested

If you're sexually active, you need to get tested for HIV and other STDs from time to time—even if you use condoms. (Remember, condoms greatly reduce your risk of contracting STDs, but they're not a guarantee.) It can be scary to acknowledge that you might have an STD. But if you're infected, it's best to know as soon as possible, so you can start getting treatment to stay healthy and avoid infecting others. It's estimated that 1 out of 5 people who have HIV don't know it.

In most places, you can get tested for free and you don't have to tell your parents.

When to Get Tested

The most commonly used HIV tests look for the antibodies your body starts to make once it's infected with HIV. It can take up to 3 months, or in rare cases up to 6 months, for your body to make enough antibodies to be detected. So if you think you've been infected, you should wait three months to get tested (and don't have unprotected sex in the meantime) or get tested twice.

For more information on HIV testing, and to find a testing site near you, visit www.hivtest.org, or call 1-800-CDC-INFO (232-4636).

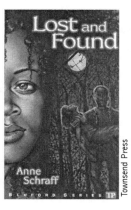

Lost and Found

Darcy Wills winced at the loud rap music coming from her sister's room.

> My rhymes were rockin'
> MC's were droppin'
> People shoutin' and hip-hoppin'
> Step to me and you'll be inferior
> 'Cause I'm your lyrical superior.

Darcy went to Grandma's room. The darkened room smelled of lilac perfume, Grandma's favorite, but since her stroke Grandma did not notice it, or much of anything.

"Bye, Grandma," Darcy whispered from the doorway. "I'm going to school now."

Just then, the music from Jamee's room cut off, and Jamee rushed into the hallway.

The teen characters in the Bluford novels, a fiction series by Townsend Press, struggle with many of the same difficult issues as the writers in this book. Here's the first chapter from *Lost and Found*, by Anne Schraff, the first book in the series. In this novel, high school sophomore Darcy contends with the return of her long-absent father, the troubling behavior of her younger sister Jamee, and the beginning of her first relationship.

"Like she even hears you," Jamee said as she passed Darcy. Just two years younger than Darcy, Jamee was in eighth grade, though she looked older.

"It's still nice to talk to her. Sometimes she understands. You want to pretend she's not here or something?"

"She's not," Jamee said, grabbing her backpack.

"Did you study for your math test?" Darcy asked. Mom was an emergency room nurse who worked rotating shifts. Most of the time, Mom was too tired to pay much attention to the girls' schoolwork. So Darcy tried to keep track of Jamee.

"Mind your own business," Jamee snapped.

"You got two D's on your last report card," Darcy scolded. "You wanna flunk?" Darcy did not want to sound like a nagging parent, but Jamee wasn't doing her best. Maybe she couldn't make A's like Darcy, but she could do better.

Jamee stomped out of the apartment, slamming the door behind her. "Mom's trying to get some rest!" Darcy yelled. "Do you have to be so selfish?" But Jamee was already gone, and the apartment was suddenly quiet.

Darcy loved her sister. Once, they had been good friends. But now all Jamee cared about was her new group of rowdy friends. They leaned on cars outside of school and turned up rap music on their boom boxes until the street seemed to tremble like an earthquake. Jamee had even stopped hanging out with her old friend Alisha Wrobel, something she used to do every weekend.

Darcy went back into the living room, where her mother sat in the recliner sipping coffee. "I'll be home at 2:30, Mom," Darcy said. Mom smiled faintly. She was tired, always tired. And lately she was worried too. The hospital where she worked was cutting staff. It seemed each day fewer people were expected to do more work. It was like trying to climb a mountain that keeps getting taller as you go. Mom was forty-four, but just yesterday she said, "I'm like an old car that's run out of warranty, baby. You know what happens then. Old car is ready for the junk heap. Well, maybe that hospital is gonna tell me one of these days—'Mattie Mae Wills, we don't need you anymore. We can get somebody younger and cheaper.'"

"Mom, you're not old at all," Darcy had said, but they were only words, empty words. They could not erase the dark, weary lines from beneath her mother's eyes.

Darcy headed down the street toward Bluford High School. It was not a terrible neighborhood they lived in; it just was not good. Many front yards were not cared for. Debris—fast food wrappers, plastic bags, old newspapers—blew around and piled against fences and curbs. Darcy hated that. Sometimes she and other kids from school spent Saturday mornings cleaning up, but it seemed a losing battle. Now, as she walked, she tried to focus on small spots of beauty along the way. Mrs. Walker's pink and white roses bobbed proudly in the morning breeze. The Hustons' rock garden was carefully designed around a wooden windmill.

As she neared Bluford, Darcy thought about the science project that her biology teacher, Ms. Reed, was assigning. Darcy was doing hers on tidal pools. She was looking forward to visiting a real tidal pool, taking pictures, and doing research. Today, Ms. Reed would be dividing the students into teams of two. Darcy wanted to be paired with her close friend, Brisana Meeks. They were both excellent students, a cut above most kids at Bluford, Darcy thought.

"Today, we are forming project teams so that each student can gain something valuable from the other," Ms. Reed said as Darcy sat at her desk. Ms. Reed was a tall, stately woman who reminded Darcy of the Statue of Liberty. She would have been a perfect model for the statue if Lady Liberty had been a black woman. She never would have been called pretty, but it was possible she might have been called a handsome woman. "For this assignment, each of you will be working with someone you've never worked with before."

Darcy was worried. If she was not teamed with Brisana,

maybe she would be teamed with some really dumb student who would pull her down. Darcy was a little ashamed of herself for thinking that way. Grandma used to say that all flowers are equal, but different. The simple daisy was just as lovely as the prize rose. But still Darcy did not want to be paired with some weak partner who would lower her grade.

"Darcy Wills will be teamed with Tarah Carson," Ms. Reed announced.

Darcy gasped. Not Tarah! Not that big, chunky girl with the brassy voice who squeezed herself into tight skirts and wore lime green or hot pink satin tops and cheap jewelry. Not Tarah who hung out with Cooper Hodden, that loser who was barely hanging on to his football eligibility. Darcy had heard that Cooper had been left back once or twice and even got his driver's license as a sophomore. Darcy's face felt hot with anger. Why was Ms. Reed doing this?

Hakeem Randall, a handsome, shy boy who sat in the back row, was teamed with the class blabbermouth, LaShawn Appleby. Darcy had a secret crush on Hakeem since freshman year. So far she had only shared this with her diary, never with another living soul.

It was almost as though Ms. Reed was playing some devilish game. Darcy glanced at Tarah, who was smiling broadly. Tarah had an enormous smile, and her teeth contrasted harshly with her dark red lipstick. "Great," Darcy muttered under her breath.

Ms. Reed ordered the teams to meet so they could begin to plan their projects.

As she sat down by Tarah, Darcy was instantly sickened by a syrupy-sweet odor.

She must have doused herself with cheap perfume this morning , Darcy thought.

"Hey, girl," Tarah said. "Well, don't you look down in the mouth. What's got you lookin' that way?"

It was hard for Darcy to meet new people, especially someone like Tarah, a person Aunt Charlotte would call "low class." These were people who were loud and rude. They drank too much, used drugs, got into fights and ruined the neighborhood. They yelled ugly insults at people, even at their friends. Darcy did not actually know that Tarah did anything like this personally, but she seemed like the type who did.

"I just didn't think you'd be interested in tidal pools," Darcy explained.

Tarah slammed her big hand on the desk, making her gold bracelets jangle like ice cubes in a glass, and laughed. Darcy had never heard a mule bray, but she was sure it made exactly the same sound. Then Tarah leaned close and whispered, "Girl, I don't know a tidal pool from a fool. Ms. Reed stuck us together to mess with our heads, you hear what I'm sayin'?"

"Maybe we could switch to other partners," Darcy said nervously.

A big smile spread slowly over Tarah's face. "Nah, I think I'm gonna enjoy this. You're always sittin' here like a princess collecting your A's. Now you gotta work with a regular person, so you better loosen up, girl!"

Darcy felt as if her teeth were glued to her tongue. She fumbled in her bag for her outline of the project. It all seemed like a horrible joke now. She and Tarah Carson standing knee-deep in the muck of a tidal pool!

"Worms live there, don't they?" Tarah asked, twisting a big gold ring on her chubby finger.

"Yeah, I guess," Darcy replied.

"Big green worms," Tarah continued. "So if you get your feet stuck in the bottom of that old tidal pool, and you can't get out, do the worms crawl up your clothes?"

Darcy ignored the remark. "I'd like for us to go there soon, you know, look around."

"My boyfriend, Cooper, he goes down to the ocean all the time. He can take us. He says he's seen these fiddler crabs. They look like big spiders, and they'll try to bite your toes off. Cooper says so," Tarah said.

"Stop being silly," Darcy shot back. "If you' re not even going to be serious . . . "

"You think you're better than me, don't you?" Tarah suddenly growled.

"I never said—" Darcy blurted.

"You don't have to say it, girl. It's in your eyes. You think I'm a low-life and you're something special. Well, I got more friends than you got fingers and toes together. You got no friends, and everybody laughs at you behind your back. Know what the word on you is? Darcy Wills give you the chills."

Just then, the bell rang, and Darcy was glad for the excuse to turn away from Tarah, to hide the hot tears welling in her eyes. She quickly rushed from the classroom, relieved that school was over. Darcy did not think she could bear to sit through another class just now.

Darcy headed down the long street towards home. She did not like Tarah. Maybe it was wrong, but it was true. Still, Tarah's brutal words hurt. Even stupid, awful people might tell you the truth about yourself. And Darcy did not have any real friends, except for Brisana. Maybe the other kids were mocking her behind her back. Darcy was very slender, not as shapely as many of the other girls. She remembered the time when Cooper Hodden was hanging in front of the deli with his friends, and he yelled as Darcy went by, "Hey, is that really a female there? Sure don't look like it. Looks more like an old broomstick with hair." His companions laughed rudely, and Darcy had walked a little faster.

A terrible thought clawed at Darcy. Maybe she was the loser, not Tarah. Tarah was always hanging with a bunch of kids, laughing and joking. She would go down the hall to the lockers and greetings would come from everywhere. "Hey, Tarah!" "What's up, Tar?" "See ya at lunch, girl." When Darcy went to the lockers, there was dead silence.

Darcy usually glanced into stores on her way home from school. She enjoyed looking at the trays of chicken feet and pork ears at the little Asian grocery store. Sometimes she would even steal a glance at the diners sitting by the picture window at the Golden Grill Restaurant. But today she stared straight ahead, her shoulders drooping.

If this had happened last year, she would have gone directly to Grandma's house, a block from where Darcy lived. How many times had Darcy and Jamee run to Grandma's, eaten applesauce cookies, drunk cider, and poured out their troubles to Grandma. Somehow, their problems would always dissolve in the warmth of her love and wisdom. But now Grandma was a frail figure in the corner of their apartment, saying little. And what little she did say made less and less sense.

Darcy was usually the first one home. The minute she got there, Mom left for the hospital to take the 3:00 to 11:00 shift in the ER. By the time Mom finished her paperwork at the hospital, she would be lucky to be home again by midnight. After Mom left, Darcy went to Grandma's room to give her the malted nutrition drink that the doctor ordered her to have three times a day.

"Want to drink your chocolate malt, Grandma?" Darcy asked, pulling up a chair beside Grandma's bed.

Grandma was sitting up, and her eyes were open. "No. I'm not hungry," she said listlessly. She always said that.

"You need to drink your malt, Grandma," Darcy insisted, gently putting the straw between the pinched lips.

Grandma sucked the malt slowly. "Grandma, nobody likes me at school," Darcy said. She did not expect any response. But there was a strange comfort in telling Grandma anyway. "Everybody laughs at me. It's because I'm shy and maybe stuck-up, too, I guess. But I don't mean to be. Stuck-up, I mean. Maybe I'm weird. I could be weird, I guess. I could be like Aunt Charlotte . . ." Tears rolled down Darcy's cheeks. Her heart ached with loneliness. There was nobody to talk to anymore, nobody who had time to listen, nobody who understood.

Grandma blinked and pushed the straw away. Her eyes brightened as they did now and then. "You are a wonderful girl. Everybody knows that," Grandma said in an almost normal voice. It happened like that sometimes. It was like being in the middle of a dark storm and having the clouds part, revealing a patch of clear, sunlit blue. For just a few precious minutes, Grandma was bright-eyed and saying normal things.

"Oh, Grandma, I'm so lonely," Darcy cried, pressing her head against Grandma's small shoulder.

"You were such a beautiful baby," Grandma said, stroking her hair. "'That one is going to shine like the morning star.' That's what I told your Mama. 'That child is going to shine like the morning star.' Tell me, Angelcake, is your daddy home yet?"

Darcy straightened. "Not yet." Her heart pounded so hard, she could feel it thumping in her chest. Darcy's father had not been home in five years.

"Well, tell him to see me when he gets home. I want him to buy you that blue dress you liked in the store window. That's for you, Angelcake. Tell him I've got money. My social security came, you know. I have money for the blue dress," Grandma said, her eyes slipping shut.

Just then, Darcy heard the apartment door slam. Jamee had come home. Now she stood in the hall, her hands belligerently on her hips. "Are you talking to Grandma again?" Jamee demanded.

"She was talking like normal," Darcy said. "Sometimes she does. You know she does."

"That is so stupid," Jamee snapped. "She never says anything right anymore. Not anything!" Jamee's voice trembled.

Darcy got up quickly and set down the can of malted milk. She ran to Jamee and put her arms around her sister. "Jamee, I know you're hurting too."

"Oh, don't be stupid," Jamee protested, but Darcy hugged her more tightly, and in a few seconds Jamee was crying. "She was the best thing in this stupid house," Jamee cried. "Why'd she have to go?"

"She didn't go," Darcy said. "Not really."

"She did! She did!" Jamee sobbed. She struggled free of Darcy, ran to her room, and slammed the door. In a minute, Darcy heard the bone-rattling sound of rap music.

Lost and Found, *a Bluford Series™ novel, is reprinted with permission from Townsend Press. Copyright © 2002.*

Want to read more? This and other Bluford Series™ novels and paperbacks can be purchased for $1 each at www.townsendpress.com.

Teens:
How to Get More Out of This Book

Self-help: The teens who wrote the stories in this book did so because they hope that telling their stories will help readers who are facing similar challenges. They want you to know that you are not alone, and that taking specific steps can help you manage or overcome very difficult situations. They've done their best to be clear about the actions that worked for them so you can see if they'll work for you.

Writing: You can also use the book to improve your writing skills. Each teen in this book wrote 5-10 drafts of his or her story before it was published. If you read the stories closely you'll see that the teens work to include a beginning, a middle, and an end, and good scenes, description, dialogue, and anecdotes (little stories). To improve your writing, take a look at how these writers construct their stories. Try some of their techniques in your own writing.

Reading: Finally, you'll notice that we include the first chapter from a Bluford Series novel in this book, alongside the true stories by teens. We hope you'll like it enough to continue reading. The more you read, the more you'll strengthen your reading skills. Teens at Youth Communication like the Bluford novels because they explore themes similar to those in their own stories. Your school may already have the Bluford books. If not, you can order them online for only $1.

Resources on the Web

We will occasionally post Think About It questions on our website, www.youthcomm.org, to accompany stories in this and other Youth Communication books. We try out the questions with teens and post the ones they like best. Many teens report that writing answers to those questions in a journal is very helpful.

How to Use This Book in Staff Training

Staff say that reading these stories gives them greater insight into what teens are thinking and feeling, and new strategies for working with them. You can help the staff you work with by using these stories as case studies.

Select one story to read in the group, and ask staff to identify and discuss the main issue facing the teen. There may be disagreement about this, based on the background and experience of staff. That is fine. One point of the exercise is that teens have complex lives and needs. Adults can probably be more effective if they don't focus too narrowly and can see several dimensions of their clients.

Ask staff: What issues or feelings does the story provoke in them? What kind of help do they think the teen wants? What interventions are likely to be most promising? Least effective? Why? How would you build trust with the teen writer? How have other adults failed the teen, and how might that affect his or her willingness to accept help? What other resources would be helpful to this teen, such as peer support, a mentor, counseling, family therapy, etc?

Resources on the Web

From time to time we will post Think About It questions on our website, www.youthcomm.org, to accompany stories in this and other Youth Communication books. We try out the questions with teens and post the ones that they find most effective. We'll also post lessons for some of the stories. Adults can use the questions and lessons in workshops.

Discussion Guide

Teachers and Staff:
How to Use This Book in Groups

When working with teens individually or in groups, you can use these stories to help young people face difficult issues in a way that feels safe to them. That's because talking about the issues in the stories usually feels safer to teens than talking about those same issues in their own lives. Addressing issues through the stories allows for some personal distance; they hit close to home, but not too close. Talking about them opens up a safe place for reflection. As teens gain confidence talking about the issues in the stories, they usually become more comfortable talking about those issues in their own lives.

Below are general questions to guide your discussion. In most cases you can read a story and conduct a discussion in one 45-minute session. Teens are usually happy to read the stories aloud, with each teen reading a paragraph or two. (Allow teens to pass if they don't want to read.) It takes 10-15 minutes to read a story straight through. However, it is often more effective to let workshop participants make comments and discuss the story as you go along. The workshop leader may even want to annotate her copy of the story beforehand with key questions.

If teens read the story ahead of time or silently, it's good to break the ice with a few questions that get everyone on the same page: Who is the main character? How old is she? What happened to her? How did she respond? Another good starting question is: "What stood out for you in the story?" Go around the room and let each person briefly mention one thing.

Then move on to open-ended questions, which encourage participants to think more deeply about what the writers were feeling, the choices they faced, and the actions they took. There are no right or wrong answers to the open-ended questions.

Open-ended questions encourage participants to think about how the themes, emotions, and choices in the stories relate to their own lives. Here are some examples of open-ended questions that we have found to be effective. You can use variations of these questions with almost any story in this book.

—What main problem or challenge did the writer face?

—What choices did the teen have in trying to deal with the problem?

—Which way of dealing with the problem was most effective for the teen? Why?

—What strengths, skills, or resources did the teen use to address the challenge?

—If you were in the writer's shoes, what would you have done?

—What could adults have done better to help this young person?

—What have you learned by reading this story that you didn't know before?

—What, if anything, will you do differently after reading this story?

—What surprised you in this story?

—Do you have a different view of this issue, or see a different way of dealing with it, after reading this story? Why or why not?

Credits

The stories in this book originally appeared in the following Youth Communication publications:

"Why Are Teens Still Getting HIV?" by Adam Wacholder, *New Youth Connections*, April 2004; "What If...?" by Anonymous, *New Youth Connections*, September/October 1995; "How HIV Works," by Zaineb Nadeem, *New Youth Connections*, April 2004; "Saying Goodbye to Uncle Nick," by Josbeth Lebron, *New Youth Connections*, April 1995; "Drunk for One Night, Scared for Six Months," by Anonymous, *New Youth Connections*, April 2004; "Why Are We Still Taking Risks?" by Orubba Almansouri, *New Youth Connections*, January/February 2009; "Keeping Quiet," by Anonymous, *New Youth Connections*, January/February 2009; "My Uncle Died of AIDS...And I Still Love Him," by Anonymous, *New Youth Connections*, December 1987; "Date With Destiny," by Anonymous, *Represent*, September/October 2006; "How Reliable Are Condoms?" by Ashley Amey, *New Youth Connections*, May/June 2002; "A Sad Silence," by Desirée Guéry, *New Youth Connections*, November 2002; "All Too Real: Teens Living With HIV," by NYC writers, *New Youth Connections*, January/February 2009; "Scared to Buy Rubbers? So Was I!" by Cassaundra Worrell, *New Youth Connections*, December 1987; "My Favorite Uncle Is HIV-Positive," by Akia Thomas, *New Youth Connections*, January/February 1994; "Fear of AIDS Killed Sarah," by Christine Boose, *New Youth Connections*, December 1990; "The Facts About HIV and AIDS," by NYC writers, *New Youth Connections*, April 2004; "Suffering in Silence," by Diane Brandon, *New Youth Connections*, January/February 2006; "Twenty Years Living Positive," by NYC writers, *New Youth Connections*, January/February 2009; "Acting Is My Activism," by Marsha Dupiton, *New Youth Connections*, January/February 2009; "My Dad Has HIV," by Anonymous, *New Youth Connections*, April 2001; "Too Big a Risk," by Anonymous, *New Youth Connections*, January/February 2009; "There's More to Sex Than Sex," by Anonymous, *New Youth Connections*, September/October 1992; "No Excuse Is Good Enough," by Mimi Callaghan, *New Youth Connections*, May/June 1998; "HIV: Still Searching for a Cure," by Courtney Smith, *New Youth Connections*, January/February 2009.

About
Youth Communication

Youth Communication, founded in 1980, is a nonprofit youth development program located in New York City whose mission is to teach writing, journalism, and leadership skills. The teenagers we train become writers for our websites and books and for two print magazines: *New Youth Connections*, a general-interest youth magazine, and *Represent*, a magazine by and for young people in foster care.

Each year, up to 100 young people participate in Youth Communication's school-year and summer journalism workshops, where they work under the direction of full-time professional editors. Most are African-American, Latino, or Asian, and many are recent immigrants. The opportunity to reach their peers with accurate portrayals of their lives and important self-help information motivates the young writers to create powerful stories.

Our goal is to run a strong youth development program in which teens produce high quality stories that inform and inspire their peers. Doing so requires us to be sensitive to the complicated lives and emotions of the teen participants while also providing an intellectually rigorous experience. We achieve that goal in the writing/teaching/editing relationship, which is the core of our program.

Our teaching and editorial process begins with discussions

between adult editors and the teen staff. In those meetings, the teens and the editors work together to identify the most important issues in the teens' lives and to figure out how those issues can be turned into stories that will resonate with teen readers.

Once story topics are chosen, students begin the process of crafting their stories. For a personal story, that means revisiting events in one's past to understand their significance for the future. For a commentary, it means developing a logical and persuasive point of view. For a reported story, it means gathering information through research and interviews. Students look inward and outward as they try to make sense of their experiences and the world around them and find the points of intersection between personal and social concerns. That process can take a few weeks or a few months. Stories frequently go through ten or more drafts as students work under the guidance of their editors, the way any professional writer does.

Many of the students who walk through our doors have uneven skills, as a result of poor education, living under extremely stressful conditions, or coming from homes where English is a second language. Yet, to complete their stories, students must successfully perform a wide range of activities, including writing and rewriting, reading, discussion, reflection, research, interviewing, and typing. They must work as members of a team and they must accept individual responsibility. They learn to provide constructive criticism, and to accept it. They engage in explorations of truthfulness, fairness, and accuracy. They meet deadlines. They must develop the audacity to believe that they have something important to say and the humility to recognize that saying it well is not a process of instant gratification. Rather, it usually requires a long, hard struggle through many discussions and much rewriting.

It would be impossible to teach these skills and dispositions as separate, disconnected topics, like grammar, ethics, or assertiveness. However, we find that students make rapid progress when they are learning skills in the context of an inquiry that is personally significant to them and that will benefit their peers.

When teens publish their stories—in *New Youth Connections* and *Represent*, on the Web, and in other publications—they reach tens of thousands of teen and adult readers. Teachers, counselors, social workers, and other adults circulate the stories to young people in their classes and out-of-school youth programs. Adults tell us that teens in their programs—including many who are ordinarily resistant to reading—clamor for the stories. Teen readers report that the stories give them information they can't get anywhere else, and inspire them to reflect on their lives and open lines of communication with adults.

Writers usually participate in our program for one semester, though some stay much longer. Years later, many of them report that working here was a turning point in their lives—that it helped them acquire the confidence and skills that they needed for success in college and careers. Scores of our graduates have overcome tremendous obstacles to become journalists, writers, and novelists. They include National Book Award finalist and MacArthur Fellowship winner Edwidge Danticat, novelist Ernesto Quiñonez, writer Veronica Chambers, and *New York Times* reporter Rachel Swarns. Hundreds more are working in law, business, and other careers. Many are teachers, principals, and youth workers, and several have started nonprofit youth programs themselves and work as mentors—helping another generation of young people develop their skills and find their voices.

Youth Communication is a nonprofit educational corporation. Contributions are gratefully accepted and are tax deductible to the fullest extent of the law.

To make a contribution, or for information about our publications and programs, including our catalog of over 100 books and curricula for hard-to-reach teens, see www.youthcomm.org.

About the Editors

Laura Longhine is the editorial director at Youth Communication, where she oversees editorial work on the organization's books, websites, and magazines. She edited *Represent*, Youth Communication's magazine by and for teens in foster care, for three years.

Prior to joining Youth Communication, Longhine was as a staff writer at the *Free Times*, an alt-weekly in South Carolina, and a freelance reporter for various publications. Her stories have been published in *The New York Times*, *Legal Affairs*, newyorkmetro.com, and *Child Welfare Watch*. She has a bachelor's in English from Tufts University and a master's in journalism from Columbia University.

Longhine is the editor of several other Youth Communication books, including *Why I'm Still a Virgin: Teens Write About Saying No to Sex* and *Analyze This! A Teen Guide to Therapy and Getting Help*.

Keith Hefner co-founded Youth Communication in 1980 and has directed it ever since. He is the recipient of the Luther P. Jackson Education Award from the New York Association of Black Journalists and a MacArthur Fellowship. He was also a Revson Fellow at Columbia University.

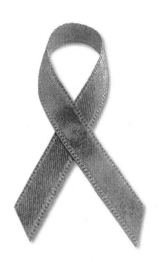

More Helpful Books
From Youth Communication

The Struggle to Be Strong: True Stories by Teens About Overcoming Tough Times. Foreword by Veronica Chambers. Help young people identify and build on their own strengths with 30 personal stories about resiliency. (Free Spirit)

Starting With "I": Personal Stories by Teenagers. "Who am I and who do I want to become?" Thirty-five stories examine this question through the lens of race, ethnicity, gender, sexuality, family, and more. Increase this book's value with the free Teacher's Guide, available from youthcomm.org. (Youth Communication)

Real Stories, Real Teens. Inspire teens to read and recognize their strengths with this collection of 26 true stories by teens. The young writers describe how they overcame significant challenges and stayed true to themselves. Also includes the first chapters from three novels in the Bluford Series. (Youth Communication)

Out of the Shadows: Teens Write About Surviving Sexual Abuse. Help teens feel less alone and more hopeful about overcoming the trauma of sexual abuse. This collection includes first-person accounts by male and female survivors grappling with fear, shame, and guilt. (Youth Communication)

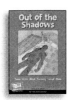

Out With It: Gay and Straight Teens Write About Homosexuality. Break stereotypes and provide support with this unflinching look at gay life from a teen's perspective. With a focus on urban youth, this book also includes several heterosexual teens' transformative experiences with gay peers. (Youth Communication)

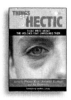

Things Get Hectic: Teens Write About the Violence That Surrounds Them. Violence is commonplace in many teens' lives, be it bullying, gangs, dating, or family relationships. Hear the experiences of victims, perpetrators, and witnesses through more than 50 real-world stories. (Youth Communication)

The Teen Guide to Sex (without regrets). Help teens understand that sex isn't something that just happens to them—they have choices. These teen writers answer common questions, and describe how becoming sexually active has changed their lives, for better or worse. (Youth Communication)

My Secret Addiction: Teens Write About Cutting. These true accounts of cutting, or self-mutilation, offer a window into the personal and family situations that lead to this secret habit, and show how teens can get the help they need. (Youth Communication)

Sticks and Stones: Teens Write About Bullying. Shed light on bullying, as told from the perspectives of the bully, the victim, and the witness. These stories show why bullying occurs, the harm it causes, and how it might be prevented. (Youth Communication)

Boys to Men: Teens Write About Becoming a Man. The young men in this book write about confronting the challenges of growing up. Their honesty and courage make them role models for teens who are bombarded with contradictory messages about what it means to be a man. (Youth Communication)

Growing Up Together: Teens Write About Being Parents. Give teens a realistic view of the conflicts and burdens of parenthood with these stories from real teen parents. The stories also reveal how teens grew as individuals by struggling to become responsible parents. (Youth Communication)

To order these and other books, go to:
www.youthcomm.org
or call 212-279-0708 x115

DEC — — 2013

CPSIA information can be obtained at www.ICGtesting.com
Printed in the USA
267991BV00006B/171/P

9 781935 552376